Yoga Wonderland

Adventures in
Self-Guided
Home Yoga Practice

Teri ALICE Leigh

MOZI Publications

Disclaimer

This book and program provides information on yoga theory, healing techniques, spirituality, and lifestyle. The author and the publisher are not licensed physicians, chiropractors, acupuncturists, or other health care practitioners, and the information in this book does not constitute a diagnosis.

This book is intended as a supplemental reference manual to complement the instruction of a qualified yoga instructor. It is not intended to replace or be used in lieu of such instruction. A qualified yoga instructor will provide specific contraindications of poses, safe alignment and sequencing of poses, and modifications appropriate for individual bodies.

More by Teri Leigh

BOOKS

MOZI Your Way to Mindfulness

30 Days of Muchness: A Mindfulness Program for Eating, Exercise, and Meditation

The Gift Inside the Wound

Yoga Wonderland: Adventures in Home Practice

The Shadow's Shine: The Summer of 1985

ONLINE LEARNING PROGRAMS

Body Wisdom: Mindfulness in Healthy Posture & Mechanics

The Goldilocks Principle: A Practical Guide to the Chakras

The MOZI Method for Mindfulness

Yoga Wonderland: Adventures in Home Practice

www.MindfulnessOnlineAcademy.com
www.TeriLeigh.com

Praise for Yoga Wonderland

"This book is a light and happy read, sprinkled with lots of pixie dust. I"

"A fascinating look at yoga practice from a different viewpoint and one that is almost revolutionary in concept."

"This practice is what we as a world need in an era of divisiveness and anxiety. Take a moment to slow your life, slow your breath, and digest this delightful book, and you'll be better for it."

"This book gives you room to reflect, the freedom to develop technique while guiding you toward your own practice that is fueled with your own insights and revelations."

"An easy read, and an easy-to-follow book that guides you to connect with yourself, and to breathe. "

"This book is not just about stretching, but about understand yourself and your daily needs."

Table of Contents

Preface

Alice's Adventures in Wonderland is a multi-dimensional sacred text that offers spiritual truths in a way that keeps me playing in Wonderland each time a read a passage. My inner-child knows how to wander through imaginary nonsensical lands and make up my own rules.

On the other hand, as a yogi, I have always found the stories of Hindu mythology far too complicated and confusing. Their epic mythologies are, well, just that, epic. I cannot relate to the carnage and dragon slaying of the *Mahabharatha*. To me, the imaginary world of a hookah smoking caterpillar and a Mad-Hatter's tea table are far more intriguing than the endless wars and battles over morality of Hindu mythology.

In 2012, I re-read *Alice's Adventures in Wonderland* (and every year since) and found myself writing copious notes in the margins detailing my thoughts about the symbolism of the creatures and characters in the novel and their parallels to concepts I learned on my yoga mat.

My 2012 yogi's log entries marked a turning point in my home yoga practice. That was the year I unlocked the tiny door to my own personal Yoga Wonderland. My practice shifted from a mundane daily to-do task to something I ABSOLUTELY LOVE AND CRAVE EVERY DAY! **YOGA WONDERLAND** is such an amazing place where every practice I discover out-of-the-way-things and where never-expected-occurrences happen. **IT. IS. SO. MUCH. FUN!!!**

Down the Yoga Rabbit Hole

Practice with Yoga Teachers

Falling Down the Yoga Rabbit Hole

Alice started to her feet, for it flashed across her mind that she had never before seen a rabbit with either a waistcoat-pocket, or a watch to take out of it, and burning with curiosity, she ran across the field after it, and fortunately was just in time to see it pop down a large rabbit-hole under the hedge.
In another moment down went Alice after it, never once considering how in the world she was to get out again.

I was nine years old when I tried my first yoga pose, not much older than Alice was when she followed her White Rabbit. My body was still limber enough to put my foot behind my head and stick my tongue out at my parents while pretending to be a turtle. Yoga was a game I played on the family room floor in the mid 1980s, looking to a simple black and white picture book as my guide. By the time I hit adolescence, I outgrew the game and shelved my copies of The Children's Garden of Yoga and Alice's Adventures in Wonderland, picking up Carrie by Stephen King and Flowers in the Attic by V.C. Andrews instead.

Fifteen years later, I fell down the yoga rabbit hole once again. My White Rabbit, masquerading as my cardio-kickboxing instructor, invited me to try her yoga stretch class that was scheduled after my favorite Wednesday night cardio-kickboxing class. Twenty minutes after punching and kicking an invisible opponent, I found myself playing like a dog, soaring like an eagle, and standing atop the world's highest mountain. I tumbled, quite literally, head over knees over shoulders, down the yoga rabbit hole. Less than halfway through that very first yoga class, I knew I couldn't climb my way back out, nor did I want to. Yoga was far more fun than right hooks, upper-cuts, and roundhouse kicks. I wasn't fighting anymore. I was playing!

The rabbit-hole went straight on like a tunnel for some way, and then dipped suddenly down, so suddenly that Alice had not a moment to think about stopping herself before she found herself falling down what seemed to be a very deep well.

For me, chasing a White Rabbit down the yoga rabbit hole was a swift fall into a lifelong passion that is now so deeply knitted into the threads of my bone marrow that it is now a part of my being.

Very quickly after my first class with my kickboxing instructor, a second White Rabbit came hopping through the tunnels. I followed that second yoga instructor to my first class in an actual yoga studio to a world where upside-down is natural, left feels like right, and backward is the same as forward.

Either the well was very deep, or she fell very slowly, for she had plenty of time as she went down to look about her and to wonder what was going to happen next. First, she tried to look down and make out what she was coming to, but it was too dark to see anything: then she looked at the sides of the well, and noticed that they were filled with cupboards and book- shelves: here and there she saw maps and pictures hung upon pegs.

Presently she began again. "I wonder if I shall fall right through the earth! How funny it'll seem to come out among the people that walk with their heads downwards!

As Alice felt the hole might not have a bottom, I wondered if the ninety-minute class might never end. Like Alice mused about the various oddities on the shelves of the rabbit hole walls, I mused about the strange atmosphere of the yoga studio: the statue of the man with an elephant head, the unique scent of nag champa incense, and the foreign sounds of Sanskrit chanting.

But most of all, I was fascinated by the *colors*.

That first yoga class in a yoga studio was like the White Rabbit took me down a tunnel that led to the yellow brick road of technicolor dream world. Perhaps it was the delirium from the over-hot room, but I remembered something else about being a child, I remembered a sight I'd had that I'd spent most of my grow-up years ignoring.

Around the time I was playing with tortoise pose on the living room floor with my parents, I discovered I had a rare ability to see auras. My parents had been taking a series of intuitive development self-awareness courses. When my dad described to my ten-year-old self that people have colors dancing around them as expressions of their moods and thoughts, I laughed and described his to him in great detail. For much of my teenage years, long after I'd given up yoga after being teased about my passion for it at summer camp, my dad and I played a different game. A game of "what color do you see." Throughout my adolescence, I practiced and developed this third eye sight as just something fun I did with my dad. But once I got to college, I put that game on the same shelf in the back of my bedroom closet with a handmade ouija board.

In that Bikram yoga class in 2001, for ninety-minutes of twenty-six poses, each performed twice, I watched a laser light show of auras beam around the room like a kaleidoscope. With each pose, the light show changed. I watched bubbles and arrows escape my instructors mouth and float around the room landing in and on the students, changing their colors into clearer images. My yoga instructor kept prodding me to look at my own eyes in the mirror, but I was having too much fun chasing the light beams through the looking glass to pay her much mind.

. . .when suddenly, thump! thump! down she came upon a heap of stick sea dry leaves, and the fall was over.

She was close behind it when she turned the corner, but the Rabbit was no longer to be seen: she found herself in a long, low hall, which was lit up by a row of lamps hanging from the roof.

There were doors all round the hall, but they were all locked; and when Alice had been all the way down one side and up the other, trying every door, she walked sadly down the middle, wondering how she was ever to get out again.

She came upon a low curtain she had not noticed before, and behind it was a little door about fifteen inches high: she tried the little golden key in the lock, and to her great delight it fitted!

What makes my tumble down the yoga rabbit hole unique to most is that while I initially followed a White Rabbit down the hole, **my rabbit**

disappeared quicker than I could follow. And finding another rabbit to follow was more difficult in 2001 than it was in 2005 or 2015 or even today. The nearest yoga studio was a two-hour drive away, and I couldn't get there more than once or twice a month. I yearned to take class every day, or even twice a day. The more I made that two-hour drive to class, the more excited and more frustrated I got.

I wanted MORE!

While I loved the classes and the laser light shows they brought to my third-eye-sight, I quickly tired of the teacher reprimanding me for looking around the room too much and not paying attention to just myself. I bored of the same monologue coming out of the teacher's mouth every class. I wanted a teacher who could explain to me what I was seeing in the auras. I wanted someone to show me the deeper spiritual wisdom of the practice.

I took class from all the teachers in the studio, and none of them had my sight, nor did they stray far enough from the prescribed monologue to offer me the spiritual insights I craved. All of the teachers I met spoke only of the mental and physical benefits of yoga. Honestly, I didn't entirely love my White Rabbit, or the couple of his friends he introduced me to. Where, oh where, would I find someone who could see what I could see AND teach me yoga?

Like Alice, and any yoga practitioner who has committed to a several-times-a-week practice, I was far beyond the point of no return. I couldn't climb back up the rabbit hole and go back to my world as it was before. I couldn't unsee what I saw. I couldn't close my third-eye and put it back to sleep again. I couldn't un-do the poses I had done, or the effect they had on my system.

I found myself without a yoga teacher, facing a hall of locked doors, and there were no other White Rabbits to be found. Besides, I really wouldn't be content chasing an occasional White Rabbit through another dark tunnel. I had to find a way through one of those doors.

If I learned anything from my childhood play in *The Children's Garden of Yoga,* I learned that there is a whole wonderland of yoga. My inner child yogi knew that no White Rabbit yoga instructor or rabbit hole class could show me the wonderland that existed on the other side of the tiny door behind the curtain.

The White Rabbit

Once upon a time, you wanted to try yoga, something you've never done before. Likely, the first thing you did was find a teacher. Like Alice's White Rabbit, your first yoga teacher took you down a dark tunnel to a place you'd never been before. She set the pace, and she sometimes got annoyed when you didn't keep up. If you did as she said, in precisely the same way that she instructed, you were sure to succeed.

but what were you succeeding at?
a complex game of follow the leader?

At some point, your White Rabbit might tell you that you learned everything she had to teach you, and either she hands you off to another more experienced White Rabbit, or she sends you to find one yourself. In time, some White Rabbit might even give you your own rabbit suit and waistcoat with a timepiece so you can become a White Rabbit yourself, teaching others what you have learned from your white rabbits.

This is how things work in the world of learning. There are teachers (White Rabbits), and courses (rabbit hole tunnels), and rules (waistcoats), and parameters (timepieces). They expect you to trust them to be your guide. They tell you what to do, how to do it, and when to do it. They explain to you why you are doing something and how it serves you in the future. They have completed extensive trainings and certification programs to hold their AUTHORITY.

The Yoga Rabbit Hole

Millions of yogis have followed White Rabbits down the yoga rabbit hole. Over the years, yoga teachers have multiplied, like . . . well. . . rabbits! As a yoga practitioner, whether you accidentally-on-purpose found yourself in a yoga class like I did, or you went sliding down the slippery slope with arms up screaming "wheeee" all the way down, you have likely encountered many different White Rabbits (yoga teacherss) along your path.

Inevitably, in any journey, circumstances change. You may lose a favorite teacher, or many teachers. Schools close. Teachers move away, or fall off their pedestals. Or, you simply grow bored because you have learned everything they have to teach you. We are conditioned through life to seek a teacher, an authority, to show us how to do things we don't know how to do. So, when we lose our teachers, the natural response is to go in search of another one. New teachers may take you down some different tunnels, but those tunnels are *their* tunnels, not *your* wonderland. I ask you, how many white rabbits have you collected as authorities on your ventures? How many tunnels have you explored with teachers as your tour guides?

Somehow after years of schooling, we lose the curiosity and wonderment that comes with childhood exploration, adventure, and imagination. When we chase and follow white rabbits, we forget the wonderment and curiosity that comes with exploring unknown territory on our own. After awhile, those tunnels start to feel confining, and those authority figures feel oppressive. And those timepieces and their pace feels really, well. . . limiting.

When you find yourself in that place where you don't have a teacher anymore, you have a choice, find another rabbit to take you down another tunnel, or find a way through that tiny door. I hope you choose door number one instead of rabbit number six, or tunnel number sixteen.

psst. . .come over here. . .let me show you. . .there's MORE!
Take a peek through this tiny door behind this curtain. . .

The Loveliest Garden You Ever Saw

You took a leap of faith when you followed a White Rabbit to teach you something you didn't know before. I'm here suggesting you take a completely different kind of leap. Stop following the White Rabbit yoga teachers (they run too fast ahead of you anyway). Don't go looking for another one. They just keep you in the darkened rabbit hole tunnels with them, following them through complex labyrinths. You can thank them for their service, honor them for the excellent foundation they offered you to accept out-of-the-way-things to happen. Then, let them hop away.

Venture on your own into Yoga Wonderland.

On the other side of the tiny door is the loveliest garden you ever saw! That garden has zillions of flowers and colors and plants and creatures unlike anything you have ever seen before. That garden has all kinds of wide open paths and trails and adventures you can follow to places that live beyond the perimeters of your wildest imagination. Heck, you can even build your own paths and trails just by imagining them yourself! In this place, there are no rules, no time structures, no parameters. You get to go where you want to go, do what you want to do, and play how you want to play. And when you do, the most amazing magic happens, you come to expect the unexpected. Here, in wonderland, you access your most infinite resource, your imagination. Once you turn that on, the possibilities within your world become limitless.

The deepest and most profound wisdoms cannot be accessed through the guidance of a guru. Those, you must find on your own.

Shutting Up Like a Telescope

But first, you have to take the initial step and get yourself through that tiny door. I know, that door looks teeny-tiny, and it doesn't make sense that you can fit your too-big-body through. I invite you, be like Alice, allow yourself to shut up like a telescope and expect "nothing but out-of-the-way things to happen."

The way to shrink yourself to a size that will fit through that tiny door is to shed your ego and get on your mat, by yourself. Turn off the podcasts and the videos, and DRINK YOUR BREATH. Do a pose. And then another. And do one more. Keep breathing, and see what happens.

When you get on your home Yoga Wonderland practice mat, you will fan yourself with the White Rabbit's tiny fan. The fan of your breath makes your ego shrink, as well as the things you think you know and all the things your White Rabbit teachers taught you to know. That's when your imagination grows. When you just get on your mat alone, you get to make-up-the-rules-as-you-go, like the Queen's Croquet Game.

Just do it. Get on your mat

Drink Me!

Practice Without a Teacher

The Loveliest Garden

Alice opened the door and found that it led into a small passage, not much larger than a rat-hole: she knelt down and looked along the passage into the loveliest garden you ever saw.

How she longed to get out of that dark hall, and wander about among those beds of bright flowers and those cool fountains, but she could not even get her head through the doorway.

I had already frolicked in Yoga Wonderland, long ago, as a child diving into the pages of *The Children's Garden of Yoga*. I knew what lies behind that tiny door. Intuitively, I knew the magic of wonder and play, and no White Rabbit or yoga studio class could give me that.

Behind that tiny door was a vast limitless land called Imagination. As a nine-year-old, Imagination is a very real place. When I went into mountain pose, I didn't just pretend, I *became* Morla, the giant tortoise/mountain in *The Never-ending Story*. When I took eagle pose, I found myself riding the Luck Dragon, Falcor. In tree pose, I gathered berries and strung bows with the Ewoks of *Return of the Jedi*. Of course, my favorite pose, rabbit pose brought me to the Mad-Hatter's tea table and the Queen's croquet match in *Alice's Adventures in Wonderland*.

But as a grown up, the tiny door was too small for me to squeeze through. I remembered what that wonderland was like, but adulting had severely atrophied my sense of wonder. I didn't believe Imagination was a real place anymore. The every day menial to-do lists of being a grown-up infected me with the serious bug that squashed my sense of wonder like a potato bug on the sidewalk.

I thought I needed a teacher to show me how, to teach me the rules, to give me the step-by-step instruction on what to do, how to do it, when to do it, and also what NOT to do. I had surrendered my imagination and wonder to an almighty power, Authority.

I was stuck. I didn't like the yoga teachers around me, they scolded me for watching my laser light show in the mirrors. Like military drill sergeants, they drew very clear lines between right and wrong and made me walk the tightrope, leaving absolutely no room for meandering into wonderment. At the bottom of that rabbit hole, facing the tiny door, I didn't want to go follow another rabbit. They weren't fun.

> *"Oh, how I wish I could shut up like a telescope! I think I could if I only knew how to begin." For, you see, so many out-of-the-way things had happened lately, that Alice had begun to think that very few things were really impossible.*
>
> *There seemed to be no use in waiting by the little door, so she went back to the table, half hoping she might find another key on it, or at any rate a book of rules for shutting people up like telescopes: this time she found a little bottle on it ("which certainly was not here before," said Alice), and tied round the neck of the bottle was a paper label, with the words "DRINK ME" beautifully printed on it in large letters.*

Like Alice found no use in waiting by the little door any longer, I found no use making the two-hour drive to take the same classes over and over again. I laid out my mat, and sat down next to it, afraid of what might happen if I stepped onto it without the guidance of a teacher. I went searching for a book of rules.

Being 2001, the days before podcasting and online video streaming, I bought a bunch of yoga books, CDs and DVDs. I left them on the floor next to my mat. I read them, highlighted them, watched the DVDs and listened to the CDs. But I didn't get on my mat. Like Alice, I was hesitant to drink the potion. Would it poison me? If I did a yoga practice alone without a teacher watching me, would I hurt myself? Would I do it wrong?

I left my mat there in the middle of my living room. It beckoned to me every day. And every day, I sat down next to it, contemplating all the unpleasant things that might happen.

> *However, this bottle was not marked "poison," so Alice ventured to taste it, and, finding it very nice (it had, in fact, a sort of mixed flavour of cherry-tart, custard,*

pineapple, roast turkey, toffy, and hot buttered toast),
she very soon finished it off.

But my mat wasn't poison.

Finally, one day I couldn't take it anymore. I stepped on the mat, pressed play on the the old cassette tape player and let a man with a heavy Indian accent tell me what to do. With several deep breaths, I sucked down the potion. I drank my breath. And it felt rather nice, and odd, and weird, and curious, and pleasant, and not-pleasant all at the same time.

"What a curious feeling!" said Alice. "I must be shutting
up like a telescope!"

After that first home practice, I too had a very curious feeling. While the practice itself was rather nice, the overall feeling afterward wasn't so nice. I felt very small. Too small.

I felt like a kid again, but not in the sense of wonderment and imagination I remembered from *The Children's Garden of Yoga*. Rather, I felt like a kid who didn't know the rules, who didn't know what I was doing. I wore out that cassette tape, playing it every day I couldn't get to a studio. But there were lots of parts of it that I just didn't completely understand. The more I practiced to the CDs and DVDs and books, the more I realized I didn't know.

After a while, finding that nothing more happened, she
decided on going into the garden at once; but, alas for
poor Alice! when she got to the door, she found she had
forgotten the little golden key, and when she went back
to the table for it, she found she could not possibly reach
it: she could see it quite plainly through the glass, and
she tried her best to climb up one of the legs of the
table, but it was too slippery; and when she had tired
herself out with trying, the poor little thing sat down and
cried.

I was small enough to fit through the door. But alas, like Alice, the key (my imagination) was still out of my reach. I couldn't play in the laser light show of chakras and auras when I was alone. So I turned away from the tiny door, and went chasing after another White Rabbit, all the way to a resort in Mexico.

My next White Rabbit took me to places I didn't think I wanted to go. I went straight from stepping over puddles of sweat (ew, gross) in the carpeted halls of a hot studio to an eight-day yoga teacher training bootcamp on the beaches of Mexico. And a bootcamp it was! This White Rabbit squeezed me through corners that weren't exactly comfortable. Some of them even hurt, a lot.

Balance on my hands in crow pose, AND jump back to plank?
Are you serious? um...okay, maybe?...
Six wheel poses, you don't need the rest in between!
Huff....Puff....I forgot HOW to breathe...Holy shit this is HARD!
Frog Pose for 30 minutes...
Owie...Ow...OW...Ouch....OUCH! (sobbing like a baby)
Now TEACH!
Um, okay. Really? I guess so...

So I taught. I put on my own White Rabbit costume and led students through the tunnels, describing to them as I taught the brilliant kaleidoscopic colors and laser lights I saw along the way. I admit, I liked playing the center of the stage, commanding a class to do what I told them, when I told them, and how I told them to do it. I felt like Mickey Mouse in *Fantasia* conducting my own armies of animals through the galaxies of colors. I enjoyed the power (and the ego that came with it) of leading a large group of people to move synchronistically, breathe simultaneously, and flow in unison. And I studied what happened. I kept a detailed log of the results that occurred in each class. I became a yoga-scientist coordinating my own mad-tea-parties.

Whenever I could, I'd go back to my White Rabbit, doing more trainings and bootcamps, practicing with him via CD and DVD every day. I got to the highest level of training and certification. Heck, I even certified many white rabbits to lead students through the same tunnels I showed them.

The longer I taught, the more the labyrinth of tunnels grew, and the more rabbits populated those tunnels. All of them wanting more and more people to follow them, and many of them wanting to train even more rabbits. Yoga teachers multiplied, like rabbits!

The more rabbits there were, the more tunnels were dug, the darker those tunnels felt to me. Too many white rabbits were becoming not just significant characters, but the main characters in the adventures.

But I wasn't the main character in anyone's rabbit hole. I was only an occasional one. Just like my white rabbits were for me, flitting through from time to time. But mostly, I just followed their mirages in the form of CD and DVD practices.

For the bulk of my yoga teaching career, I traveled across America, guest presenting. I sprinkled my fairy dust insights in a studio space for a week or two, and then ventured off to another place. Some students would continue to follow me (my mirage), virtually, via my podcasts. Others waited for me to return once or twice a year.

The rabbit holes got more crowded, and yet I still couldn't find a rabbit who could see what I could see or teach me what I wanted to learn. I always walked away from class with a longing. A deeper craving that couldn't be filled by another class. I kept coming back to the tiny door, but it couldn't be unlatched by any podcast or video, other teacher, master class, specialty workshop, or intensive training.

Ultimately, all the classes and teachers said the same thing.

The answer lies within.

"Come, there's no use in crying like that!" said Alice to her- self rather sharply. "I advise you to leave off this minute!"

She generally gave herself very good advice (though she very seldom followed it), and sometimes she scolded herself so severely as to bring tears into her eyes; and once she remembered trying to box her own ears for having cheated herself in a game of croquet she was playing against herself, for this curious child was very fond of pretending to be two people. "But it's no use now," thought poor Alice, "to pretend to be two people!

Why, there's hardly enough of me left to make one respectable person!"

I had to give myself my own advice, and (gulp) take it. I couldn't look to someone else to be my guide. I couldn't pretend to be a White Rabbit for everyone else, and also be the one chasing white rabbits of my own. Pretending to be two people was no longer of any use to me. I had to be myself, just me, and my home practice was the only way to teach myself how. I had to be my own teacher.

Soon her eye fell on a little glass box that was lying under the table: she opened it, and found in it a very small cake, on which the words "EAT ME" were beautifully marked in currants. "Well, I'll eat it," said Alice, "and if it makes me grow larger, I can reach the key; and if it makes me grow smaller, I can creep under the door: so either way I'll get into the garden, and I don't care which happens!"

The cake had been there along, my yoga mat unrolled in the middle of the living room, just patiently waiting for me to put away the CDs and DVDs. The mysterious wonders of my imagination and my inner child self did not exist in the words of a yoga teacher, or within the walls of yoga class with other students. While I could see hints of it there, just like Alice could see the garden through the tiny doorway, I couldn't really experience the wonders of the garden until I got on my mat by myself, without the guidance of a teacher. To limit myself to class with a teacher was to stay at the bottom of the rabbit hole and never venture beyond the tiny door behind the curtain.

She ate a little bit, and said anxiously to herself "Which way? Which way?", holding her hand on the top of her head to feel which way it was growing; and she was quite surprised to find that she remained the same size. To be sure, this is what generally happens when one eats cake; but Alice had got so much into the way of expecting nothing but out-of-the-way things to happen, that it seemed quite dull and stupid for life to go on in the common way. So she set to work, and very soon finished off the cake.

So I ate. At first I took tiny little nibbles. And then larger bites. At first nothing out-of-the-way seemed to be happening. So I kept eating. When I committed to finishing the whole cake, that's when the magic really started happening.

What I realized in my first efforts at a solo home yoga practice was that turning within myself, looking to myself to be my own teacher was like shutting myself up like a telescope to see the truth inside myself. This is what yoga is all about. A telescope is used to see (*scope*) far away (*tele*). Turning the telescope in on myself is to see far inside myself!

So now, I step alone on my mat and turn in on myself at least five times a week. My home yoga practice is my adventure through that wonderland on the other side of a tiny door into the loveliest garden I have ever seen.

It was all very well to say "Drink me," but the wise little Alice was not going to do that in a hurry. "No, I'll look first," she said, "and see whether it's marked 'poison' or not'"

Alice's drink didn't have a list of ingredients or nutritional information. She didn't know what side effects she might experience. Just as Alice is hesitant to drink the potion, I suspect you are also rather hesitant about practicing alone. I promise you won't shrink to the size of a mouse, nor will you "get burnt and eaten up by wild beasts or other unpleasant things." Practicing alone is not poison, but rather, it is an enlightening elixir. It is a process of wonder and curiosity.

I invite you to join me in this grand and mysterious garden with your own taste buds as your tour guide. Drink the potion and eat the cakes. Swallow the ones that taste good, and spit out the ones that don't. See what unexpected things happen.

As with any program, you get out of it what you put into it. In order to fully experience the wonders of Yoga Wonderland, you need to commit to yourself and your practice. I hope that you keep it small and simple, especially in the beginning. Can you give yourself just five minutes a day? Just five minutes a day and you will access some of the most powerful wisdoms that live inside yourself. If you commit to five minutes, you'll find yourself craving and wanting more.

*Commit to
5-minutes a day,
5 poses a day,
5 breaths a pose,
for 5 days a week.*

What You Will Learn

Access Your Imagination

*"Imagination is EVERYTHING.
It is the preview to life's coming attractions."
~Albert Einstein*

Should you choose to drink the potion and commit to this Yoga Wonderland Program you will unlock the tiny door to the mysterious wonders of your inner-child self, and tap into your most abundant and infinite resource, YOUR IMAGINATION. The more you practice, the more out-of-the-way-unexpected things will happen. You will remember the joy and play of a child exploring new lands.

And one day, I hope, your Yoga Wonderland, as mine did for me, will start to spill itself like colored sand and glitter into the every day workings of your normal life. The greater life lessons you explore on your mat start to highlight themselves with rainbow twinkling in your day-to-day occurrences. When that happens, everyday life can no longer be dull and boring. Rather, it becomes a kaleidoscope of adventures in the people you meet, the places you go, the things you do, and the feelings you feel.

By the end of the program, I hope your imagination opens up wide like mine did. Perhaps you will even allow yourself to become a unique character who contributes to the curious world of Yoga Wonderland.

Be Your Own Teacher

"The answers lie within ourselves. If we can't find peace and happiness there, it's not going to come from the outside."
~Tenzin Palmo

Without a White Rabbit as a tour guide, every day in Yoga Wonderland is a challenge of your ego to look inside yourself rather than look to an authority. When you step onto your mat without the guidance of a teacher, you force yourself to be your own teacher.

The characters in Alice's Wonderland are the teachers that live inside yourself. They never offer Alice direct answers to her questions. Rather, more often than not, they answer her questions with more questions, always turning the discovery process back to her.

If you let the characters of Alice's Wonderland serve as your mentors, or better yet, as your own voice talking to you, they challenge you to ask yourself more questions. They will inspire you to be curious, to open your mind to wonder, and to dig deep inside yourself to find your own answers.

Listen to Your Body

"When you listen to your body when it whispers,
You will never have to hear it scream." ~Unknown

When a teacher is telling you what to do, you ears are too full of your teacher's words to hear the quiet whispers of your own body. But, when you practice alone, the soft wise voice of your body gets loud. When you step onto your mat without a teacher, you are forced to pay attention to the language of your body as it tells you what to do, how to do it, and where to go next.

While Yoga Wonderland does offer you a simple sequence of (about) five poses per module, it does not offer any instruction on alignment or modifications. This lack of instruction is intentional because yoga poses are not stock one-size-fits-all for every body. Everyone has certain poses that just don't work in their bodies. And, everyone has poses that work really well in their bodies.

In addition, every day the poses manifest differently than the day before. Some days your body may feel strong and solid, while other days it is more flexible. Some days you may feel balanced, while other days you feel creaky and tight. Sometimes you feel big, and other times you feel small. Yoga Wonderland challenges you to pay attention to these shifts and changes and to respond accordingly. No one can tell you what is best for your body because you are the only one who can feel it.

Ultimately, in our every day lives, it is easy to go about doing and experiencing things without ever really paying attention to how your actions really feel in your body. Yoga Wonderland is your time every day to move, pause, and listen to what your body is saying with each action (or inaction). Yoga Wonderland teaches you how to be body aware.

Discipline

> "We are what we repeatedly do.
> Excellence, then, is not an act,
> but a habit."
> ~Aristotle

When you commit to doing something everyday, and make it a repetitive habit in your life, it becomes a practice. That practice becomes progress. Progress creates change. When we do something simple, in repetition, over and over, it becomes our reality.

One of the greatest magical side effects of this program is the activation of discipline in your system. Discipline of doing small things many times as part of your every day routine effects the most drastic and powerful changes (for the better) in your world. You will find that once you commit to this program and it becomes a part of your natural life habits, discipline toward other things in your life will evolve as well.

Why You Should Practice Alone

Whether you are a seasoned yoga practitioner, a trained and certified yoga teacher, or relatively new to this mystifying and magical practice, you somehow followed a white rabbit down a yoga rabbit hole and found yourself in a world where upside-down is natural, inside out is outside in, left feels like right, and backwards is the same as forwards. In taking classes at studios, studying with teachers, or going through workshops and trainings, you have explored a labyrinth that exists down the yoga rabbit hole.

You Want MORE

There comes a time in every yogi's practice, given you have been practicing somewhat consistently (if even just a couple times a month) when you will hit a plateau. Yoga studios and classes offer a slew of workshops, trainings, and teacher trainings to "take your practice to the next level." You can spend thousands of dollars (or tens of thousands) on further training, and you will likely still hit another plateau.

But, there is one level of the practice that no workshop, seminar, training, or certification program can offer. That level comes with the commitment to practice alone on your mat without the guidance of a teacher. And if you commit fully to that level of practice, a self-guided personal practice, you may never have to experience a significant plateau in your practice again. (I certainly haven't).

If you pay attention, every yoga teacher, class, workshop or training will tell you that ultimately the answers you seek lie within yourself. Yoga is a practice in turning within to find those answers. But, if you are listening to a teacher tell you how, that teacher is holding you back from the ultimate expression of your own answers and truth, because their voice is not, and cannot ever be your own still small voice within. Once you access that still small voice within, and really listen to it, its wisdom is limitless. The still small voice inside you has a lot to say, so much that you will never run out of new things to learn and experience on your mat again.

I suggest you let the white rabbit hop along without you. Step onto the looking glass of your yoga mat. Shut yourself up like a telescope and turn in on yourself. Unlock the tiny door behind the curtain to the most glorious YOGA WONDERLAND that can only be found by practicing alone, without a teacher.

Save Time & Money

Studying yoga with teachers is expensive, both in your money and your time. Yoga is a very expensive hobby. But it doesn't have to be.

According to a recent study examining yoga trends and habits of over 2,000 Americans was conducted by OnePoll and Eventbrite, dedicated yoga practitioners will spend on average $1044 a year on yoga classes. Add to that expense the additional costs of apparel, equipment, workshops, and trainings, the average committed yogi will spend upwards of $34,000 in yoga in a lifetime.

At the same time, the average yoga student claims that taking a regular one-hour class can eat up an average of 2-3 hours a day. By the time they get dressed and packed for class, drive to class, take class, drive home, and get showered and changed, yoga takes up a good chunk of your day. If you practice 4-5 times a week, your time commitment to yoga can be anywhere from 8 to 15 hours a week. This does not count the additional time spent for longer workshops and intensive trainings.

In 2018, when I retired from teaching yoga, I conducted a personal statistical analysis of my practice cost in time and money. As a small business owner, I keep track of my yoga expenditures as business write-offs each year. I also keep track of my time spent on the mat in my yogi's log journal. From my first tumble down the yoga rabbit hole to date, I have spent over $75,000 and 40,000 hours, resulting in a per year average of $4400 and 2,350 hours.

After retiring from teaching, I committed 100% to my Yoga Wonderland home practice. I now spend on average 20-30 minutes on my mat, 5 days a week, totaling 2.5 hours a week. Because my practice is at home, there is no time spent commuting, arriving early to get my spot, or staying late to socialize. My total financial investment is no $0.

What's most intriguing to me, however, is not the statistics of numbers of hours or cost in dollars, but rather the notes in my yogi's journals. When I flip through my journals since November 2018, the insights, excitements, ahas, and expressions of joy have multiplied exponentially! While I am practicing less, and spending nothing, my experience of the practice is the best it has ever been!

Yoga Teaching

I taught yoga full-time for nearly fifteen years. In that time, I took thousands of classes from hundreds of teachers nationwide. I trained and certified hundreds of teachers myself. What I have come to understand in my experience is that without a doubt, the absolute best teachers are the ones who are committed to a self-guided home practice. Within just 3-5 minutes of any class I take, I can tell by the energy and aura of the teacher whether they are committed to their own self-guided home practice.

The number one problem yoga teachers face is burn-out. Almost every teacher, at some time in their career, sacrifices their own practice for their teaching. When they do, their teaching tanks. As yoga teachers, our time is limited because (like most teachers) you are running all over town to teach too many classes a week for not enough income and managing a home and family, and possibly even a day job, you simply don't have the leftover 2-3 hours a day to get on your mat in a class.

When burnout happens, you lose your love and passion for the practice, and you have nothing left to share with your students. Your teaching becomes mundane. Your voice becomes a monotonous parrot of quotes and overdone cues you have heard, used, and recycled in hundreds of classes.

As a yoga teacher, you absolutely MUST practice what you teach in order to effectively serve your community. It's simple. If you aren't practicing, your teaching loses its power. The ONLY way to combat teacher burnout is to practice. Take care of yourself and your own needs before giving to your students or you will suffer depletion. Self-guided home practice makes battling teacher burnout even easier because you are not strapped by the conditions of time and expense.

If you commit to a home practice, your skill and impact as a teacher will improve exponentially. Most yoga teachers do not have a home practice. Therefore, if you commit to a home practice, you will significantly set yourself apart from the vast sea of multiplying White Rabbits in the yoga rabbit hole tunnels. Because you will be teaching the insights that you discovered inside yourself on your own, your classes will present a fresh perspective, a completely authentic voice, unique cueing based on what you have felt in your own tissues, and creative approaches that are not available in the recycled classes taught by everyone who is teaching what everyone else teaches. Your class sizes will increase, and your students will rave about your wisdom and insight more than you ever knew possible.

Alice in Wonderland

Perhaps you are drawn to this program for no other reason than because you love Lewis Carroll's *Alice's Adventures in Wonderland*. The beloved children's story is timeless, and its wisdoms are abundant and true. Even if you aren't a huge fan of yoga, perhaps you just love reading interpretations of this sacred spiritual text to discover the deeper meanings hidden inside the nonsensical wonderland. Please, come play with me in Yoga Wonderland and let the Cheshire Cat, the Mad Hatter, the Red Queen, and the Moral Duchess be your new insightful friends.

Your Yoga Wonderland Mentor

Teacher vs Mentor

I changed my title from teacher (authority) to mentor (peer). My job as mentor is to encourage you to be your own teacher, to listen to your own insights, and discover things on your own, in your body, and in your heart that no one else can show you. I am vigilant that I will NOT tell you what to do or when to do it. I'll only share with you little tea-cup tidbits I have found in my wonderland, all the while, encouraging you to break any and all rules you've ever had to follow.

Mentorship is a simple game of questions, and curiosity, and more questions, and more curiosity. And encouraging you to bite the tootsie pop and chew the gooey center. My goal as your mentor is to help spark more questions, to trigger more curiosity. Along the way, I'll show you some of the things I figured out without the help of a teacher or instructor. But moreso, I'm hoping YOU will show ME and everyone else in the program, the wonder-filled things that YOU discover without a teacher telling you how. And hopefully, somewhere amidst all those questions and explorations and adventures and discoveries, you'll find yourself smack dab in the middle of your most infinite resource, your IMAGINATION!

Eat Me!

Un-Learning with Un-Rules

TERI LEIGH

Eating the Cakes

At the end of Chapter I of *Alice's Adventures in Wonderland,* Alice makes a decision to eat the cake and see what happens. If you have gotten this far into this program, perhaps you, like Alice, have decided to eat the cake, commit to the process of a solo home yoga practice and see what happens next.

But, eating the cake means precisely that, you don't know what is going to happen next. You are willing to bite into something new, chew it, swallow it, and let it digest and metabolize into your system. In doing so, you are going to change the chemical make-up of your body, mind and spirit. Buckle your seatbelt! You are in for an adventure into the center of your Self like you have never had before.

When I look at the running-backwards-timepiece that I smashed long ago, it's "hindsight is 20/20" time-keeping tells me that I wasted a lot of my Yoga Wonderland play-time by pounding on that tiny door begging for the rulebook to show me how to get through. I would have been much better off just biting into the cake, swallowing the first bite whole, and going along for the ride instead of requiring that I knew all the rules and expectations beforehand.

THERE ARE NO RULES!

But first, I went looking into the adventures of other people's home yoga practice programs. I did podcasts, and videos. I even worked my way through a number of workbooks that promised *40 Days to. . .* and *Six-Week Program for. . .* Every podcast, video, workbook, and only program had instructions and directions. Some of them had so many dos and don'ts that I couldn't keep up.

Do this. Don't do that. Do it this way. Don't do it that way.
Do this after that, but don't do that after this. Change.

With each one, I asked myself, "what is the use of a home practice to look inside myself when someone else is telling me what to do and think?"

*Rules and instructions are
the murderers of adventure and curiosity!*

Yoga practice, whether on podcasts or videos, or in studios and with teachers, feels like a complex process with a zillion little rules to remember and apply, dozens of them for each pose. Add on top of that a vast library of *sutras* including complex teachings such as the *yamas* and *niyamas,* and yoga becomes something too overwhelming to even try in the first place. When done with a class or instructionally guided home-practice, I often felt like my creativity had been decapitated like a dandelion was victim to school-child singing that grotesque rhyme "mama had a baby and got it's head chopped off" while flicking the fuzzy yellow top off its stem with her thumb.

So, as your not-white-rabbit, I hand you this key to your wonderland. The key fits when you throw away all the rules, drop what you think you may know, and un-learn what you have been taught. When you do this, you allow your inner child-like sense of curiosity and wonderment to thrive. The only rules in wonderland is that there are no rules!

The very nature of a world without rules means that there isn't any application process, or pre-requisite list, or proof of mastery of skills you must provide to gain entry. The *only* requirement is that you BELIEVE.

*Believe in the magic.
Believe in your imagination.
Believe in yourself and your ability
to make things up as you go along.*

And the way to believe, to Make-Believe, is the simplest and hardest part of the whole venture. It's simply getting on your mat and doing a stretch, and taking a breath, and another breath, and maybe another stretch. That's it. Even if you have never ever done a single yoga pose in your life before, you can get into wonderland if you believe you can do a breath and do a stretch. But, that stretch has to be the way YOU make it up to be, not how any White Rabbit has ever said it should be. In Yoga Wonderland, you are not allowed to *should on yourself,* because *shoulding* on yourself is the quickest one-way ticket back to the world of darkened rabbit hole tunnels, or worse, hearing the Red Queen proclaim "OFF WITH YOUR HEAD!"

When I finally did get through the tiny door, I did it by creating my own rule-book. Actually, it's an un-rule book.

These un-rules are five things I had to un-learn about myself and my approach to yoga and life. They are five feathers I had to pluck out of my hat and leave to be trampled on by other rabbits in the rabbit holes. In actuality, they are rather opposite of what you might expect.

I gotta be honest with you, I've broken every single one of them *many times,* because, well, I forget, or I get lazy, or that day I just don't seem to care. That's called being human. And every time I forget, the Red Queen of Hearts threatens to decapitate my ego-head like a dandelion, killing all sense of curiosity and wonderment.

I invite you to block the Red Queen of Hearts and all her nonsensical rules and concepts, replace her with your inner-child's most abundant resource, IMAGINATION!

Un-Rule #1
The Rule of Fives

The first step into Yoga Wonderland, is also the hardest step. Just practice. It sounds so simple. Yet, it's so dang hard to do. For me, when I finally committed to practice without a teacher, my ego dropped on the floor with a thud and I found I had shrunk like a telescope to a size that will fit through that tiny door.

Practice at home and practice in classes are two entirely different creatures. At a studio my practice is follow-the leader, surrender-to-the-teacher, and play-off-the-energies-of-the-other-students. A studio practice is a work-out, carefully crafted long sequence designed to work every muscle, joint, tissue, and organ, taking into account the rise to a peak pose, a surrender to a deep pose, and so much more. Alone, my practice is be-my-own-boss, listen-to-myself, and build-my-own-energy-inside-myself. A home practice is a work-in, exploring my body and my feelings and sensations, listening to what I feel and how I think. If I expected to get out of practice at home what I got out of practice in classes, nothing at home worked or felt right. If I tried to find the feels in a class that I found in my home practice, they played hide-and-seek with me, only they had really good hiding places. In time, I realized that applying my studio practices to my home practice was a massive motivation killer.

When I tried listening to podcasts or watching video streamed classes, I found myself having these full-on angry dialogues with the teachers inside my head.

I don't want to do that pose now.
Dang, that's a stupid thing to say.
Would you just stop rambling already?
Slow down, I wasn't ready to get to that cue just yet!

After awhile, I found myself turning-off or tuning-out the podcast and doing my own thing. That's when the practice became fun. That's when I entered wonderland. So for awhile, I tricked myself into getting into wonderland by starting practice by following the hologram of a white rabbit in the form of a podcast, and then ignoring the hologram entirely so I could go into Yoga Wonderland. I needed a way to be motivated to practice without the white rabbits, without the holograms. In order to do that, I had to drop my prior conceptions of practice. That's when I made up my Rule of Fives.

The Rule of Fives
Cheat Sheet

5-Minutes

I only have to get on the mat for 5-minutes. Any more than 5-minutes is bonus. If I hit 5-minutes, I can count this as a practice.(Pretty much always, I want to stay longer than 5 minutes.)

5-Poses

If I do a total of 5 poses, I've succeeded. It doesn't matter which 5 poses, or the order in which I do them, I just need to do FIVE. (I usually start with child's pose, and I usually do more than five.)

5-Breaths

I hold each pose for at least 5-breaths before I can call it complete. The longer and slower and deeper and more even the breaths, the better. (5-breaths is usually 30-seconds, and I usually hold longer.)

5-Days a Week

I give myself two days to skip, because well, stuff happens. Besides, even God rested once a week. Yet, 5-days is still most days. (I noticed, the day after a skip day is usually AWESOME!)

Bonus

If I get as far as 5-minutes, 5-poses, 5-breaths, or 5-days, I consider myself solid. If I do more than FIVE of any or all of these, BONUS! (and guess what? I am BONUS-ING all the time!)

Un-Rule #2
Breath First

Every yoga teacher in the world will tell you that the most important aspect of practice is breath. "Breathe" is probably one of the most commonly uttered cue in any yoga class. We all have heard it, probably thousands of times out of the mouths of yoga teachers everywhere, both in classes and on podcasts. And, as good follow-the-leader students, we listen, and follow, and breathe every time we are told. Yet, we forget. And forget. And forget yet again.

In yoga classes, teachers tell me to prioritize my breath, but every time a teacher tells me to do something else, I focus on that, and forget about breathing. And then she'd tell me to breathe. But then I would forget about whatever physical cue she had just given so I could breathe. Evidently multi-tasking is not my strong suit.

The first time I actually spent the WHOLE practice paying attention to my breath didn't happen in a class with a teacher. It happened during a phase in my home practice when the majority of my practice was sun salutations.

My favorite teacher had once suggested I try a set of ten consecutive sun salutation Bs doing every movement on one breath. The first several times I tried this, I caught myself trying to catch my breath by halfway through the set. Of course, this made me think that I was extremely out of shape. When it wasn't getting any easier after nearly two weeks, I figured I had to be doing something wrong. And then, one morning, something miraculous happened. I got on my mat feeling particularly heavy after a rather sleepless night. I just couldn't push myself, so while I still committed to doing ten sun Bs, I had to slow them down, a lot. By the third one, I noticed something drastically different was happening.

Instead of my breath keeping up with my body, my body was following my breath. As I inhaled, my torso felt like it was inflating, floating up. And as I exhaled, I felt everything deflate, surrender, get pulled down. I literally felt like my breath was making my body move, and everything was EASY! Before I knew it, I had floated through not just ten, but over a dozen sun salutations, without once losing my breath or pace. I fell into a cadence and rhythm that was driven by how my breath fed my heartbeat.

After somewhere between 15 and 20 sun salutations, I paused in mountain pose, and literally felt like I was both on top of the mountain and embodying the mountain at the same time. It was one of those magical unexpected moments on the mat that I will never forget. I not only intellectually understood the concept of breath being important, but I also *embodied* it. I became the essence of breath. It was almost as though I could feel the higher infusion of oxygen in my bloodstream. I was high on my own breath!

I continued to move through a full-practice, feeling into almost every pose I knew, breath leading me. I got into arm balances and binds that I had never been able to access before. Backbends and shoulder openers that I had only before experienced as painful felt more than good. They felt great! I held poses for longer, enjoying them more. I lost track of time, and played in this new Yoga Wonderland space for what turned out to be over four hours. And, I wasn't sore the next day!

From that practice forward, every single pose I do starts with breath, and the action of my body parts follow in a sort of cause and effect. My practice continued to slow down as my breath found a depth I didn't know possible. It was also around this time that I became addicted to my home practice, craving it, anxious to hit my mat every day. I even went a solid year without going to class without even really missing the studio classes at all. And miraculously, my fitness level didn't decline. when I did go back to a class, it was physically easier!

Within the span of a month or so another magical thing happened, I realized everything I was doing *felt really good*. We all know that post savasana yoga bliss feeling that happens. Well, multiply that by at least ten, if not a hundred, and apply it to every single pose! Every teacher had always told me that breath was the most important, but it wasn't until I practiced alone that I really understood what that meant.

Un-Rule #3
Feel Good

Everything, absolutely EVERY. SINGLE. THING. we do on our mats MUST FEEL GOOD. If it doesn't feel good, we won't want to do it, and it'll make us stop wanting to come to our mats. We need our yoga mats to be a place that is so inviting, so enticing, so yummy-goodness-wonderful that we can't wait to get there.

Yoga Wonderland must always FEEL GOOD!

One reason for this is because when we do things that feel good, our body spills out a hormone called dopamine, which gives us a rush of happy. Let's face it, life is hard, so we need as much chemical help we can get, and not in the form of medicinally prescribed pharmaceuticals. Dopamine is a healthy internally produced hormone that brings us happy from the inside out.

A second reason to feel good in everything on our mats (*c'mon now - do we really need reasons to feel good?*) is to make sure we don't hurt ourselves. This requires dropping what we may have learned in yoga classes, particularly those that are fitness based. Teachers often say things like "feel the burn" or "breathe through it" or "the pose doesn't start until you want to leave it." These are all the yogis version of the old fitness adage "no pain no gain." In hindsight, I realize that *all* my yoga injuries happened in classes where I listened to things like this. However, I *never* get hurt when I practice alone. At home, I believe that if it feels good, especially that kind of feel good where I don't want to stop doing it, then, I'm doing it right.

One of the hardest lessons I learned in my home practice was that Yoga Wonderland is NOT my workout. I say this with all kinds of love in my heart for you, dear yogi. Let me say it again, so it settles in. Yoga Wonderland is NOT your workout. Yoga Wonderland is not your time to build your muscles and increase your flexibility, and challenge your endurance. If you make these your *goals*, you are missing the whole point, to turn INSIDE.

Trust me. I did that for far too long.

Every single time I put fitness as my focus, the Red Queen of Yoga Wonderland kicked my pretty little ego head out that tiny door with her pointy little boot, effectively exiling me from the adventures until I checked my ego at the door. Trust me on this one, squeezing a big stupid ego head out that tiny Yoga Wonderland door is not comfortable. It hurts. Usually it comes in the form of some nasty injury that forced me off my mat for longer than I was happy. There was a time in my life where I was doing ninety-minutes of Power Vinyasa Yoga in 105 degrees heat and 85% humidity every single day, sometimes twice a day, both in classes and at home. (Yes, I even built a heated studio in my house). You name a common, and even uncommon yoga injury, and I've had it. Yoga butt? yup. Knee ligament strain? uh huh. Hamstring pull? yeppers. Wrist pain? check. Shoulder ache? of course. The list goes on. It hurts.

I'm not saying fitness and physical well-being won't necessarily happen. Rather, they are likely to occur naturally as a *side effect*. By definition, a side-effect is something that happens accidentally, unintentionally, without effort. I promise you this, cross my heart, when I quit *trying and efforting* in my yoga practice and traded the fitness-focus for the feel-good-focus, I found health like I never knew possible. I finally got through the tiny door. . . and WOWZER! Now, I do 20-40 minutes of whatever gentle feel goodness my happy little body wants, and I feel better than ever. Last week I moved a heavy sofa bed up and down two flights of stairs without hurting my back. This winter, I shoveled heavy snow for two hours without losing my breath or feeling sore the next day. And, I'm ten years older than I was in those power vinyasa ego days!

Keep it simple for yourself. Only do what FEELS GOOD. If it feels good, do it. If it doesn't feel good, don't do it. ALL. THE. TIME. NO. MATTER. WHAT.

Un-Rule #4
Be Mindful

If I'm perfectly honest, Un-Rule #3: FEEL GOOD means absolutely nothing if we don't know what *good* feels like. Un-Rule #4: BE

MINDFUL is about paying attention and listening so we understand what GOOD feels like. Be Mindful is my nice way of saying to myself, "get your head on straight girl and pay attention!"

Sadly, we all run around life sometimes with our heads disconnected from our bodies. Heck, I do that *all the time*. I'm a natural born klutz, which means I am the type of person who discovers a bruise or cut on my body several days *after* it happened and can't remember how I got it because I'm being too mind-LESS to pay attention to where my my body ends and the door frame begins or to bother to remember the injury as it happens. *Sigh.*

Even though the human brain is functionally incapable of true multi-tasking, I like to pretend I am really good at it. In reality though, I can only do one thing at a time. Sure, my left hand can rub my belly while my right hand can pat my head, and it may seem like I'm multi-tasking. But in reality, my left hand is only doing one thing, rubbing my belly. And my right hand is only doing one thing, patting my head. My right hand cannot pat my belly and rub my head at the same time. And anytime I try, I get the tasks and the body parts all confused anyway.

Every yoga class I have ever taken, on some level or another, was a big game in trying to multi-multi-task. (*yes, I meant to say multi-twice*). Some instructors would give a laundry list of six, or seven, or even eleven or twelve cues in every single pose! Unable to really effectively do them all at once anymore than the instructor could spit the words of instruction out all at once, the whole thing always turned into a game of trying to keep up with machine-gun-fire directions. I always failed miserably.

Now that's not to say that I didn't find teachers who slowed down. I eventually learned to watch my students' bodies and give them one cue, and wait until they did it before giving them a different cue. There are definitely yoga teachers out there who give instructions slowly, one at a time. And, even they typically give at least three or four different things to do, one after another, in each pose. But even with only three or four cues, I still didn't have time to listen!

It was just TOO MUCH!

What I discovered when I finally landed my little bum on my mat alone in Yoga Wonderland was that I could do ONE THING, and then spend some time with my breath feeling the feels. Oh those feels felt GOOD! I took things on my own timing, and my timing was slower than a snail's or caterpillar's pace climbing a mountain. My own timing is REALLY SLOW!

For me, slowing down is the key to being mindful. Being mindful is how I learned to PAY ATTENTION. Rather than playing catch-up and keep-up with the teacher and all their cues and directions, I found I was playing follow-the-feeling, and listen-to-the-sensation with my body.

Ahhhh.

Un-Rule #5
Expect the Unexpected

These un-rules have a sort of domino effect. while un-rules 1-4 are things you can actively DO, number five is a result, something that happens as an effect of setting the right conditions with un-rules 1-4. When I put rules 1-4 in place, my practice becomes a moving meditation, where amazing and unexpected things I couldn't even plan come to happen.

I have now come to expect the unexpected to happen on the mat, and that has become the most exciting thing about my home practice. Every day, I step on my mat with a sense of wonder.

What am I gonna learn or experience or feel today?

Let me offer you an example. Once, feeling particularly dense and heavy, I got to my mat and collapsed in child's pose. I honestly thought that was all I would be able to do that day. Feeling particularly tight in my shoulders, I knew I wanted thread the needle pose, but I felt even too heavy (or lazy) to come up to my hands and knees, much less raise my arm up to the sky. And then, the unexpected happened. I discovered a new pose. I tucked my elbow under my child's pose body, turned my cheek to the floor, and let my shoulder collapse to the floor.

Ahhhh. Bliss.

While laying there with my cheek pressed against the floor, I felt like a baby with my face on my mama's chest, Mother Earth's breast. It felt SOOO GOOD! My lazy version of thread the needle, which was a hybrid of child's pose and fetal position was something I never expected to happen, and has now become a staple in the beginning of almost every practice. That first day, I stayed in infant pose for several minutes each side. It felt so nurturing to my dense and heavy body. After nearly ten minutes, my breath deepened, and I felt so supported that I eventually *wanted* to push up onto all fours. I don't remember what happened after that, but it didn't matter, I'd discovered a new pose that I had never seen in any books or been taught in any class. It became my go-to pose for those days I felt vulnerable, weak, dense, heavy, lonely, fatigued, worried, anxious, confused, overwhelmed, and well, the list goes on.

My point in this story is that every single day that I get on my mat alone, when I consciously practice the first four un-rules, something magically unexpected happens.

The Ultimate Un-Rule: Do Whatever You Want

All these traditional rules and un-rules can be boiled down to one simple concept: Do whatever you want. In wonderland, anything goes. Like a child playing make-believe, you get to do whatever you want. You get to be whomever you choose. In wonderland, there are no rules except the ones YOU create. And since it is YOUR wonderland, you get to break those rules anytime you want, and make new ones, and break the new rules too. When it comes down to it, when you do something that you want to do for yourself, the ONLY approach that works is to do it YOUR WAY.

One of my most favorite scenes in a children's movie is the final scene of *The Never-ending Story.* A child princess holds in her hand, a single grain of sand, the only remaining morsel of the magical land of Fantasia. She explains that the way to rebuild the land is to imagine it, and it becomes real again. Wonderland works the same way. In order to explore wonderland, you must first create it. The best way to create it is to make it up for yourself. The only way to do this is to do whatever you want, your way. When you do this, you automatically follow all the un-rules, breaking the walls and limitations given to you by white rabbits, teachers, and instructors of your world.

I hope that as you venture through Wonderland, creating your own world as you go along, you rediscover the kid-ness inside you. You will remember the vast abundance of your imagination. And, you will capture the ability to transform the mundane dullness of your every day life into into curious characters and adventures of your own personal wonderland.

Cheat Sheet
Yoga Wonderland's Un-Rules

Take Five
5-Minutes, 5-Poses, 5-Breaths, 5-Days-a-Week

Breath First
Everything starts with Breath

Feel Good
Everything should Feel Good.

Be Mindful
Pay Attention and play Follow-the-Sensation

Expect the Unexpected
Magic Happens on the Mat

Do Whatever You Want
Your Mat. Your Rules. Your Way.

Journal Reflections

Yoga Wonderland Un-Rules

Date:

What "rules" of yoga have never set right in me or my body?

If I could make my own rules (or un-rules) what would I make up for my own practice?

Other Thoughts/Insights?

Yoga's Yamas & Niyamas

Patanjali's *Yoga Sutras* are generally accepted as the scriptural text for yoga. In it, Patanjali outlines eight-limbs of yoga. Two of the limbs the *yamas* (moral restraints) and *niyamas* (moral observances) are considered the ten commandments of yoga, similar to the ten commandments of the Bible. Like all scriptural writings, the *yamas* and *niyamas* are subject to personal interpretation. In the theme of Yoga Wonderland, I offer here my own wonderland interpretation of these *thou shalls* and *thou shalt nots*.

Yamas - Moral Restraints

Be Kind (Ahimsa)

Yoga Wonderland is a safe space to encourage, support, and affirm. If you get mean (or hurt yourself), the Red Queen will threaten to chop off your head (ego).

Be Truthful (Satya)

Welcome to your seat at the Mad-Yoga-Hatter's table. Be true to your our own unique version version of madness AND you will find yourself curious and open to the madness in others.

Be Balanced (Brahmacharya)

Eat from BOTH sides of the hookah smoking caterpillar's mushroom. Be open to perspectives that are not your norm as that's where unexpected things happen.

Be Giving (Asteya)

The Moral Duchess seeks the meaning in everything. We all have wisdom inside us to give. Yoga Wonderland is a place to find YOUR own personal inner wisdom. Don't steal insights and wisdoms from others. Find your own.

Be Generous (Aparigraha)

The more you share, the bigger the Cheshire Cat grins. Your voice matters in Yoga Wonderland, let yourself sing.

Niyamas - Moral Observances

Be Pure (Sauca)

When standing on the witness stand bearing evidence in your trial in front of the Red Queen, the house of cards could come tumbling down if you aren't authentic and true.

Be Content (Santosha)

It's best to find contentment in anything and everything you do in Wonderland. Whiners & complainers are sent to the Red Queen.

Be Passionate. (Tapas)

Alice was determined to stand for what she believed, yet also passionate about exploring all she didn't know or understand. Be like Alice. Be passionate about every part of your experience.

Self-Study. (Svadyaya)

Alice didn't have a personal tour guide. Home yoga practice that is SELF-GUIDED is where the magic happens.

Surrender (Ishvara-Pranidhana)

In Yoga Wonderland, we have come to expect that unexpected things happen, as this is where the best wisdoms fall out of the sky. It's best to be open to all kinds of oddities and curiosities here.

Journal Reflections

Yoga Wonderland Yamas & Niyamas

Date:

In creating your own Yoga Wonderland as a place you crave to explore, what 'thou shalls' and 'thou shalt nots' do you want to hold for yourself?

Other Thoughts/Insights?

TERI LEIGH

The Loveliest Garden

Create Your Own Wonderland
Your Sacred Practice Space

Step One:
Get On Your Mat

Give your yoga mat a home. This can be as elaborate as building a separate yoga room into your house, or as simple as laying out your mat at the foot or side of your bed. I've done both.

When I first started a home practice, I was blessed to have a basement bedroom in my home that I outfitted with a special heater and stocked with an extensive prop closet. I hired a mural artiste to paint a metallic OM symbol on the wall. I installed an elaborate ancestor shrine, and created a fairy garden outside the window. I lined the walls with stones and crystals I had gathered over several years. I loved that room and the energy it held.

And then, my husband divorced me to become a monk. He got the house and the yoga room. I packed my life into my Prius and traveled the country for five years, essentially *homeless*.

While I never wanted for a place to lay my head every night, I did travel from place to place, sleeping in over 100 different beds in the course of one year. My yoga mat went everywhere I did. Unrolling it at the foot of the bed, wherever that was, became as habit as unpacking my toiletry kit in the guest bathroom and plugging my phone charger in next to the bed. I loved some of those bedside mat-homes far better than my elaborate yoga room I shared with my ex. One guest bedroom where I stayed housed the family's Halloween decorations, so my practice was inspired by witches and black cats. Another guest bedroom had a giant window looking over a north-woods Minnesota lake, so my practice was serenaded by loons. And believe it or not, I discovered that practicing in the tiny hallway leading to the bathroom of a hotel room offered an opportunity to use walls on both sides for leverage and balance.

I have unrolled my mat for practice in hundreds of gorgeous places, including a beautiful mountain view lodge, an epic ocean view Mexican palapa, the clay-mud of the Badlands of South Dakota, creek-side deep in the wooded hiking trails of a Wisconsin nature preserve, and backyard fairy cottage tiny home. Of all the hundreds of homes my mat has found, my favorite of all time is my current yoga home, a long-narrow storage closet smack in the middle of my upstairs duplex apartment.

I call my current home *the treehouse* because the front windows all look out over a rather large maple tree. Smack in the center of the *treehouse* is a long narrow storage closet with one shelf and clothes rod at the far end. This is now my *Yoga Hollow*. To some it may seem claustrophobic, as it is only 2-3 inches wider and 2 feet longer than my mat. To me, my *Yoga Hollow* is PERFECT. I use the walls on both sides as leverage to push and pull myself deeper into stretches, or as a lean-support on those days where balance isn't my best friend. It is a cozy little den where I can shut out the world, and closing the door is like closing myself up like a telescope.

My point here is that the size of the space you use doesn't matter as much as actually having a space. I find that when my mat is unrolled, particularly in a place where I see it, it calls to me. If I didn't unroll the mat as part of my unpacking in a new guest bedroom, I was far more likely to skip my practice. If I rolled up and put away my mat in the yoga prop closet, I was less likely to come back to it. But now, it stays unrolled in my yoga hollow, and it begs me to come play on it. I actually miss it on the days I skip practice.

Whether you choose to leave your mat along the side of your bed so you can literally roll out of bed onto your mat in child's pose, or clear out a portion of a closet, or remodel your sun-room into a yoga room, **find a space where you can unroll your mat, and leave it there most of the time. A space where you yoga energy can gather. A place your mat can call home.**

Step Two:
Honor Your Teachers

Our white rabbits are vital to our growth and learning. First and foremost, they showed us down the well into the rabbit hole tunnels. Secondly, they helped us to navigate through the dark and confusing places. Our white rabbits are the mythical creatures that take us to mystical places and show us magical things.

Every single thing you have ever experienced in the presence of a white rabbit, be it a yoga instructor or any other type of teacher, is woven into the fabric of your being and has become an essential part of your essence. It's important to honor not just your yoga teachers, but ALL your teachers, your mentors, your elders, and anyone who has guided you on your path. They are an essential part of the process. Every inspirational quote, every pose alignment cue, every hands-on adjustment, and every encouraging smile is threaded into the loom of your neurological memory banks. Neurological wiring LOVES TO GROW and expand like a universe, ever-evolving and spiraling outwards, begging to be activated and re-activated and put to use in any circumstance of your life. The more your neurological wiring grows, the bigger your imagination gets. The more you exercise your imagination, the larger your neurological network becomes. The inner circle spirals of ideas and concepts inform and push the outer spirals of wisdom and imagination to reach further.

As you step through the tiny door and venture into practice on your own, you need the wisdom of your white rabbits whispering in your ear. You need those voices to echo inside your head, encouraging you, affirming you, reminding you that they taught you everything you needed to know to navigate this terrain alone.

In my home practice, my own teachers' voices ping-pong inside the echo-chamber of my head, bubble-popping between my ears, and sometimes even sending electric-shock shivers down my spine. I'm not just talking about my yoga teachers. On my mat, I feel and remember the encouragements from my high school Latin teacher telling me the stories of the confidence of famous orators. I listen to my synchronized swimming coach reminding me to smile. I see my grandfather Edgar showing me the power of precision and my grandmother Florence advising me on the benefits of patience. I see the sparkle of pride in my great-aunt's eyes at my piano recitals.

Every teacher we ever have leaves an activated tattoo on our soul. There are two types of tattoos. Those that live inside the complex ladder of our DNA, bringing with them ancestral wisdom and insight passed from generation to generation. For example, every experience my grandmothers ever had, and the insights they gleaned from those experiences live inside my DNA, and work to inform my choices and behaviors. The second kind of tattoo comes from those who leave imprints on our cellular memories. Every person who ever offered me a moment that created a sensation or emotion and insight left a mark that triggers whenever that insight might be helpful to me.

In the absence of a white rabbit, we rely on our ancestral wisdom and our unconscious cellular memories to be our Wonderland tour guides. In my home yoga practice, the first thing I do is invoke these wisdoms that live inside my being.

In my practice, I activate and honor my teachers and mentors and elders by maintaining an altar to them. It's an elaborate shrine. In I have pictures of these people, items they owned, notes they wrote to me, notebooks from the classes I took from them. Heck, I even have the red dress my grandmother wore for many Christmas dinners.

But remember, there was a time when I didn't have a home and I couldn't install a shrine for my practice. And there are days now when I practice away from home, away from my hollow. Sometimes I carry just one item with me, and sometimes I just speak a name or quote or phrase at the beginning of my practice. The point is, I take a moment to ignite, turn-on, activate, or ignite the memories and wisdom from them that live inside me.

Step Three:
Focus Your Intention (Journal)

In yoga we often refer to *drishti* as the vision, or gaze. We are taught to keep our eyes still and our vision focused. For me, my yogi's adventure log, my practice journal, is my drishti. It's my intention, my focus, and the revealed perception of my reality.

I have kept journals ever since I was a little girl. Dream journals. Poetry journals. Personal journals. And yes, yoga journals. Lots of yoga journals. For yoga teacher training with Baron Baptiste in 2004, I brought a checkbook sized journal that I kept under the top corner of my mat during practice. Afterwards, I would frantically scribble everything I could remember from the practice. I left that bootcamp having filled that journal and promptly bought another, and another, and yet another. By the time I attended a 5-Day *Flowing Through the Chakras* retreat with Seane Corn two years later, I had filled several journals from various workshops and trainings. As I started teaching, I kept journals of what I saw in my students, things I was surprised that came out of my mouth, assists that I tried on and students enjoyed, and much more. For awhile even, my journals were colored pencil drawings trying to capture the images I saw in my students auras during class and analyses of their chakra adjustments. Journals from trainings and workshops and my teaching were far easier to keep and fill than the ones for my ow practice.

At first, I tried to keep elaborate journals on my practice, planning out full class sequences, scribbling and changing as happened, and then writing out detailed descriptions of insights and sensations. But those extensive home practice journals never kept long. I'd always feel too rushed, too busy after practice to take that kind of time to log everything.

And then I realized my yogi's log should be as tiny as the checkbook sized journals I favored. Rather than elaborate paragraphs and musings like I kept in my personal journal, why didn't I try just writing the main ahas, the simple take-aways. When I started doing that, my yogi's logs took on a whole different energy.

The first day I found myself reaching under that corner of my mat from pigeon pose, I wrote down something very profound, at least the writer in me thought so. When I have a thought, and I take the time to push that thought down my arm to form letters onto a page, the thought becomes more than just an idea bouncing around in my head, it becomes a feeling in my body, and then it becomes words on a page. When I loop back to re-read my journal entries, no matter what they are, I realize that many, if not all my thoughts that I wrote down become some kind of reality. While those things I don't write down usually go poof into thin air.

My practice log is very simple. I write down what I want to make real. And if I can name it in just one word, it has that much more power and energy to become real. Less is more. Then, I practice. I don't consciously come back to my drishti intention during practice. I just move, and feel, and see what happens.

After practice, I reach under that corner of my mat for my checkbook sized notebook, and I scribble down the sequence I did, or at least a short series within the practice that felt particularly significant. Then, I look back at the one word intention I wrote at the beginning. I kid you not, every single time I re-read that intention, and compare it to the sequence, a brilliant aha happens. It may be something simple, or it may be something very profound. Then, throughout the rest of my day, that same message inevitably pops up everywhere.

On those days that I don't practice, or I choose not to write in my yogi's adventure log, I don't have that beautiful gold thread of insight weaving through my whole day. I miss it. And that brings me craving my time on the mat the next time I get there. That little golden thread of insight has become one of my greatest motivators to get on my mat often.

What I know is this. When I take the time to write down my intention and my insight, in as few words as possible, that intention becomes an insight that becomes a reality of my life. I've included a template of my journal entries in the next few pages. Should you like my template, I have included a blank journal page for you to use and at the end of each module in this workbook.

Yogi's Log Journal Entry

Date/Time:

I like to include both the date and time to track patterns in time of the year as well as times of the day for practice.

Mood

> Body -
>
> Mind -
>
> Spirit -

I write down just a few words or phrases to identify how I feel or what I need going into practice.

Intention

I write down just a few words or phrases to describe what I want or need to change or shift by the end of practice.

Practice Summary

I describe here what I did in practice. Often, it is a list of the poses and sequence, but it can also be a summary of how I did practice (i.e. lots of use of the block or wall, focus on twists, focus on breath moving body, etc.)

Insight

What is the AHA or Take-Away…what did I feel or learn that I want to remember through my day?

Sample Journal Entry

Date/Time: 8.21.19 5:45am - 6:30am

Mood

Body - dense, heavy, lethargic, sluggish
Mind - stagnant, foggy
Spirit - stuck

Intention

get unstuck, find the next first step, move forward

Practice Summary

Very deep long slow breath, slower than ever sun sals, flowing from one pose to the next with breath, not stopping to hold anything, but rather blending all movements together

Insight

When I feel stuck and heavy, the answer doesn't live in a jolt to push boulder out of a resting spot, but rather, like water, breathing gently and slowly, like rain eroding the earth bed below the boulder until it shifts out of its spot. This is what **surrender** is about. It's not giving up, it's giving in to let the process unfold. slow sun sals and flowing movement with breath makes that happen.

Blank Yogi's Log Journal Template

Date/Time:

Mood

      Body -

      Mind -

      Spirit -

Intention

Practice Summary

Insight

Step Four:
Invoke the Wisdom (Prayer)

*"If there is just one thing I have learned from yoga in all my years it is that prayer is always always **always** ALWAYS answered. It may not be answered in the timing you like, or with the message you want to hear, but Spirit answers every prayer ever uttered. Every single one." ~Seane Corn*

I wrote this down in my practice journal after attending a workshop with Seane Corn at the Midwest Yoga Conference. If I pull a memory of my study with Seane Corn to the front of my mind, I can hear her voice invoking a prayer clear as day as if she were sitting next to me. Seane has a gift in her ability to invoke Spirit through prayer. Her verbal intentions that open and close practice still pluck chords in my nervous system over a decade later.

I have been praying in some form or another my entire life, from my childhood of Lutheran Sunday School, Bible School, and summer camp, to grown-up weekend retreats in shamanism, and everything in between. However, I didn't fully understand the concept of prayer until I took it to my Yoga Wonderland home practice. Prior to my yoga practice, prayer for me was just floating thoughts or recitations in my head, or awkward talking to my dead ancestors. Yoga made prayer real for me because it involved not but an embodiment of those concepts in my muscles, bones, tissues, and especially my NERVES.

I have come to understand that spirituality is actually an activation and changing and alchemical transformation of the function of my nervous system. When I feel something, and feel it deeply, my body responds differently, activating all the cellular memories in my tissues, sending and receiving and growing messages through the complex neurological wiring of my brain and spinal cord. Any sensation, touch, smell, taste, sight, sound, and especially a combination of all of them can function to create a shift in my experience. When I become mindful and aware of these sensations and I control them through intention, yes PRAYER, I can manifest the reality I want in my body and therefore my experience.

As I said earlier, I must honor all my teachers as being a part of my and collection history of my experience. In addition, I must honor all my memories, all my feelings, every single experience of my life as the collective wisdom of my being. That includes the collective wisdom of every experience of all my ancestors as well.

My shaman work taught me that prayer is answered when it is spoken with the most feeling and emotion. In order for the ancestors to hear us, we must drum up the most emotion. When I applied this concept to my home practice, it made perfect sense.

Almost every spiritual tradition I have studied uses similar methods to invoke Spirit. They light candles, and or incense, or some other fragrant smelling form of fire. They use prayer beads, or rosaries, or malas. They repeat mantras, or chant scriptures, or speak prayers.

While spiritual traditions have rather elaborate means of activating and invoking spirit, what I do before practice is, like everything else in my practice, very simple. I light a candle and a stick of incense. I look up at the giant monstrosity of a portrait of my grandfather, and I say "Hi Grandpa. what've you got to tell me today?" Sometimes, instead of Grandpa, I talk to Grandma, or my great aunt. And on days I'm feeling particularly owly, I say GiggleBumps, which is the nickname my life partner uses for God. I like the smell and feel of smoke lingering in the air around me as it feels like whatever Spirit I called in is embracing me, and eventually absorbing into me through my skin.

And, if I'm fully honest, on the days I'm feeling rather desperate, or angry, or hurt, or lost, I allow myself to be just those things, and I yell. I emote. I sob. I scream. I bang my fists on my mat and I demand that they talk to me. And then I hear Seane Corn, "prayer is always always always answered." I am always surprised, and not surprised. By the end of practice, every single time, I feel better. They (they being the collective wisdoms I have inside myself) answered my prayer in some way shape or form, if even to say, "yeah, this sucks, and you can handle it."

Step Five:
Breathe

I spent well over a year of my home practice focusing on sun salutations and how I moved with breath through them. Some of the most profound wisdoms about practice and life came to me during that year of sun sals. I spent the entire year being mindful, paying attention to how my breath moved my body from pose to pose in flow. During that year, I learned alignment, but not by studying. Rather, my breath just pushed my body into precise alignment, and I learned it as a side effect.

My journals during that time logged a large library of alignment AHAs I had never heard in classes or from teachers, as well as a vast collection of understandings about my body mechanics and chemistry. When I started teaching these concepts to my own classes, students came to me commenting that they had never felt poses, nor understood alignment and energy like that before.

Full mindful breath creates optimal alignment!

When I would breathe fully and deeply, I would inflate my body, fueling it with oxygen rich blood, and everything just sort of landed in the right and perfect place! My body responded to breath like one of those inflatable characters at a used car dealership. When I inhaled just, I found perfect posture!

Being the curious researcher that I am, I tumbled down a different kind of rabbit hole, reading the research of pulmonologists, cardiologists, respiratory therapists, neurologists, and more. I became an armchair expert on the element of oxygen and its function in the human body, and started developing my own theories about oxygen and energy based on concepts such as Caesar's Last Breath (a theory that states that at any given moment every human on earth is breathing an atom or element that Caesar exhaled in his dying breath).

Let's all agree that breath is the vehicle on which your life-force travels. Without breath, we are dead. We need breath, and more specifically, the oxygen within your breath, to fuel all the functions of your body.

In yoga, breathing practices are called *pranayama*. In Sanskrit, *prana* is the life force of the body, as symbolized by breath; *yama* literally translates as "restraint" or "death," or "surrender" and loosely translates to "control." Thus, the practice of *pranayama*, is this oddly opposing practice of controlling your breath as a means of surrendering to your life force. If that isn't upside-down, backwards and inside-out like wonderland, I don't know what is! Yet, I after my year of sun sals focused on breath, I totally get it. When I control my breath, and surrender to my breath as the vehicle that moves my body, MAGIC!

For me, the kind of breathing I did, which I call *focused breathing* (similar to *ujjayi)* moves air through my sinus cavity, which is close to the middle of the skull. Physically, this is where the ear canals, eye ducts, nasal cavity, and throat meet—and where the five senses merge. One of my major yogi's log AHAs was when I realized that my *focused breathing* activates my "sixth sense" because it is actually combines all five senses together as one. Not only did it physiologically transport oxygen through my system in the most efficient manner, it brought me to a fuller awareness of my intuition through the merging of all your senses.

If anything, I hope you have learned the importance of breath, and its ability to help you do ANYTHING better. Breath is the baseline for EVERYTHING you do in life.

While focused breathing is what works for me personally, I've discovered in working with many clients over the years that developing your own form of deep breathing, however that works for you, is fine, better even. Again, shuck the white rabbit and their how-tos (including mine), and do what feels best for you. Just Breathe deeply, however that works, and see what happens for you.

There are so many different variations of deep breathing. Some people like to breathe in through the nose and out through the mouth. Others like to breathe in, hold, and breathe out slower than you breathe in. Yet others like to work on deep belly breathing, which is quite different than my focused breathing technique of focusing on big rib expansion.

It doesn't matter how you breathe, what does matter is that you DO breathe. Especially while moving, and exerting, it is so easy to forget to breathe, hold your breath, or ignore the breath and it gets shallow.

Breathing is something we do unconsciously, all day, every day. And more often than not, we stop breathing, hold our breath, and end up catching our breath without ever realizing we had stopped in the first place. It is virtually the *only* automatic functions of the body that is vital to survival, yet we can control it. So, in essence, control of the breath, and moreso, AWARENESS of the breath is key to higher awareness of life and optimal health and wellness.

I challenge you to make CONSCIOUS BREATHING a part of your every day. When I assign my clients to practice focused breathing several times a day, they all report that breathing is the single most effective and life-changing exercise they have ever done.

Your homework is to BREATHE, 5-10 focused breaths (whatever that means to you) many times a day. If you breathe mindfully when you don't need it, you'll find yourself breathing fully when you DO need it without having to remind yourself to do so. Below are a few hints as to how to make focused conscious breathing a part of your every day life.

- 10 breaths before you get out of bed (even after naps)
- 5 breaths every time (the whole time) you wash your hands
- 1 breath every time you open an app on your phone
- 10 breaths before you go to bed
- breathe deeply while waiting at stop-signs and stop-lights
- put a "BREATHE" post-it note on common things you use
  - toilet flusher
  - your kitchen faucet
  - your bathroom mirror
  - your car steering wheel

Breathe deeply many times a day, being conscious and aware of how you are breathing.

Off the Mat Trick
Focused Breathing

Step One
- Place one hand on your ribcage and one hand on your belly.
- As you breathe deeply, make your ribs move the most.
- Keep you belly as still as possible.

Step Two
- Breathe through your nose. Mouth closed.
- Create a slight constriction at the back of your nose/throat.
- Start by "snoring" and then back off the snoring.
- Keep a slight tickle or rattle in the back of your nose/throat.

Step Three
- Make your inhalation and exhalation even.
- Slow down your breath to a slow steady rate

Dosage
- 10 breaths when you wake up
- 5 breaths while washing hands when you go to the bathroom
- while walking long hallways
- whenever you feel stressed
- 10 breaths when you go to bed

Cheat Sheet
Create a Sacred Space

Step One - Give Your Yoga Mat a Home

Put your mat somewhere that it can stay unrolled. It will call to you.

Step Two - Honor Your Teachers

Build a small altar or shrine to your ancestors and teachers whose wisdom is collectively gathered in your DNA and cellular memory.

Step Three - Focus Intention (Journal)

Keep a yogi's log or journal to document your focus, intention and insights your gathered in your practice.

Step Four - Invoke the Wisdom (Prayer)

Call in the collective wisdom through some symbolic action such as: light a candle, burn incense, ring a bell or chime, chant a mantra, or speak a prayer.

Step Five - Breathe

Being breathing, deep focused breath, and remind yourself to start initiate every movement and facilitate every action with BREATH FIRST.

Journal Reflections

Creating Your Sacred Space

Date:

Describe your sacred home yoga practice space. What about it draws you to come to it often? What is your prayer and invocation process?

Other Thoughts/Insights?

Who In the World Am I?

The Home Practice Identity Crisis
Four on the Floor Poses

Opening Like a Telescope

"Curiouser and curiouser!" cried Alice (she was so much surprised, that for the moment she quite forgot how to speak good English). "Now I'm opening out like the largest telescope that ever was! Good-bye, feet!" (for when she looked down at her feet, they seemed to be almost out of sight, they were getting so far off).

At the beginning of Chapter II, Alice feels very lost and alone. Her White Rabbit has hopped away, and she doesn't have anyone to show her what to do or how to be. The rabbit hole isn't such fun and adventurous anymore, rather it is somewhat scary now that she is all alone. She has decided to try something new, go someplace she has never gone, and the world she has entered is nonsensical and strange to her. She drank a potion that made her shrink. Then, she ate a cake that made her grow. The odd circumstances around her have changed who she knows herself to be. She begins to question her identity.

I'd be liar if I told you that my home yoga practice was always wondrous adventures of play and curiosity. Like Alice, it was all kinds of fun, except when it wasn't. Once I found myself alone on my mat without a teacher, I had my own identity crisis. And, I have to admit, I let myself wallow in it longer than I probably should have. I realized much later that I was attached to who I thought I was *supposed to be* and how the yoga practice was *supposed to look* rather than who I really am and what the yoga practice meant to me, both psychologically and physically. Both on my mat and in my life. I didn't know who I was, what I was doing, how to do it, or where I fit. I had to face every one of my own insecurities by myself. I felt very lost. Like Alice, Yoga Wonderland often created a sort of identity crisis.

The poses often felt foreign, odd, weird, and often downright impossible. More than once a practice, I felt like my body was betraying me because it wasn't doing what I thought it was *supposed to do*. Or worse, I pushed it too hard to do what I thought the pictures in the books and teacher's instructions described, I injured myself.

For the first several months of my home practice, every self-doubt ping-pong-ball bounced through my head into full-on arguments with myself.

"I don't know what I'm doing."
"Well then, make it up until you do know what you're doing."

"I'm not doing this right."
"who says there has to be a right and wrong way?"

"Why does wheel pose hurt so bad?"
"if it hurts, you don't have to do it."

"What am I doing wrong?"
"what does wrong even mean?"

"I just wish I could find a teacher."
"your best teacher is right here."

Poor Alice! It was as much as she could do, lying down on one side, to look through into the garden with one eye; but to get through was more hopeless than ever: she sat down and began to cry again.

Ultimately, when I didn't know what to start with or where to go next in my practice, or what else to do, all my teacher's voices echoed like a cacophony in my head.

"if you feel overwhelmed, take child's pose."
"if you need a break, take child's pose."
"when you find yourself out of breath, take child's pose."
"child's pose is always there for you."

Child's Pose was something I figured I could do right most of the time. Even on those days when I thought I wasn't doing it right, something about putting my head down made me stop caring or thinking too much about it anyway. Child's Pose was safe. So I did it (and still do it) often. I mean A LOT. To this day, I still use Child's Pose, every practice. Usually it is at the beginning of practice, but often it comes at unexpected times as well. Whenever I feel lonely, tired, overwhelmed, lost, bored, anxious, or anything that is inside-out or upside-down or twisted-away-from goodness, I collapse into Child's Pose. And somehow, after a few deep breaths (or a lot), I feel safe. I feel safe enough to keep going.

Alice took up the fan and gloves, and, as the hall was very hot, she kept fanning herself all the time. . .

The White Rabbit's fan represents air (breath). Alice stops crying and breathes in the fullness of her situation. As yogis do, Alice is breathing in the present moment. Still in Child's Pose, between, and after, and sometimes instead of the crying, I breathe. I drink my breath. A LOT. the combination of Child's Pose and Deep Breathing makes me feel safe. Once I feel safe, it is okay to start exploring what it is like to be me, and just me. Just as Alice does, eventually I emerge, and start again, reminding myself to practice with the innocence, openness, and adaptability of a child, the beginner's mind.

"Dear, dear! How queer everything is today! And yesterday things went on just as usual. I wonder if I've been changed in the night? Let me think: was I the same when I got up this morning? I almost think I can remember feeling a little different. But if I'm not the same, the next question is, 'Who in the world am I?' Ah, that's the great puzzle!"

Pushing up and out of Child's Pose, I get into the present moment and get curious again. And my curiosity leads me to push away from the ground, onto my hands and knees (still close to the ground for stability), into other poses that emerge from the base pose of Child's Pose: Tabletop, Cat Pose, Cow Pose, Thread the Needle. All of these poses push me away from Mama (earth), but not too far away. They urge me towards the ultimate goal of getting onto my own feet, remembering how to stand and walk on my own, my way. They also all allow movement of my spine, exploring different articulations of how my back body can move, and how it feels when I move it in different ways. Curiosity pushes into wonderment, and that builds my imagination.

5-Minute Practice
Four on the Floor

I am SAFE & SUPPORTED.
When I feel safe, I can just BE ME.
I take things STEP-BY-STEP on my own timing.

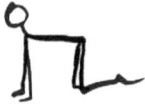 Child's Pose

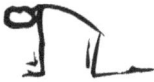 Tabletop Pose

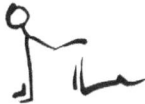 Cat Pose

Cow Pose

Thread the Needle

Child's Pose

ASANA

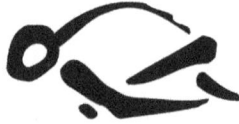

INTENTION

Everything is OKAY.
I am safe.
I am supported and grounded.
I am perfect, exactly as I am.
I accept myself.
I love myself.

Tabletop

ASANA

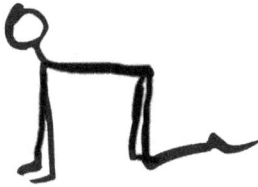

INTENTION

I am even and steady.
I can take things step-by-step.
When I take one step at a time I do less to receive more.
I can share the responsibility with all involved parties.

Cat Pose

ASANA

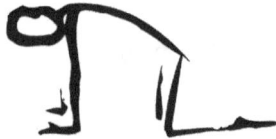

INTENTION

I have healthy boundaries.
I am self-sufficient.
I trust myself and my intuition.
I am protected.
I always land on my feet.

Cow Pose

ASANA

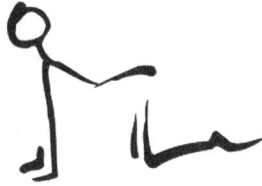

INTENTION

I am stable enough to handle scarcity.
Everything I need is provided.
I am open to receiving abundance.
The grass is green and lush everywhere.
What I give away comes back to me in abundance.

Thread the Needle

ASANA

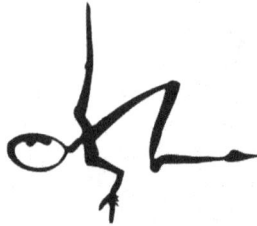

INTENTION

My body and spirit are threaded together.
I am strong, even while relaxed.
I am of both Heaven and Earth.
I am loved and supported by Mother Earth and Father Spirit.

Off the Mat Trick
MOZI Method - MULA to Feel Safe

How to Treat Anxiety & Worry in the Moment

Benefits
ASANA - improved balance and stability
INTENTION - feel safe and secure while decreasing worry & anxiety
SPIRIT - stand up for yourself

ASANA - MOVE (MULA)
- Stand with feet hip-width apart and straight like #1s.
- Evenly distribute the weight on your feet
- Soften your knees
- Feel your weight in you bum (use the "mass of your a$$")

INTENTION - THINK
- "I am safe & solid."
- "I stand on my own two feet."
- "I am balanced and stable."
- "I stand up for myself."
- "I root down to rise up."

SPIRIT - BREATHE
Breathe out while you root down into your feet. Breath out while you grow taller, reaching the crown of your head to the sky.

Dosage
Practice this for 20-50 breaths a day, both when you need it and when you don't.
- 10 breaths when you get out of bed
- 3 breaths every time you stand at a counter
- 5 breaths anytime you feel unsafe, unstable, or pushed-over
- 10 breaths before getting into bed

Four on the Floor
Journal

Date/Time:

Mood

      Body -

      Mind -

      Spirit -

Intention

Practice Summary

Insight

The Pool of Tears

Feeling Your Feels
Sun Salutations

Swimming in Tears

*Her foot slipped, and in another moment, splash! she
was up to her chin in salt-water. Her first idea was that
she had somehow fallen into the sea...*

*However, she soon made out that she was in the pool of
tears which she had wept when she was nine feet high.*

Once Alice has cried enough, she finds herself swimming in her own tears. The pool of tears represents Alice's overwhelming emotion. This symbolic purification allows her to float on the waves and motions of her emotions. She feels her feels and swims in them. She surrenders to her vulnerability, becomes completely raw and open to who she really is deep inside herself. The salt-water of her own tears washes away her fears and worries, allowing her to accept that things are different now. She is able to be consumed by the weirdness of wonderland, and to pay attention to how she engages with it.

I cannot count how many times over the years I have collapsed into Child's Pose in tears over something that has happened in my life and changed my entire world. Yoga doesn't allow me to run away from the feels, but rather offers me an opportunity to feel them, and feel somewhat safe while I feel. After a good bout of crying, and breathing in poses like child's pose and cat/cow, I always eventually get up to my feet. By the time I am standing in my first mountain pose, I am ready to wash away my feels and move on. At that point, like Alice, I find my body is swimming in the hormones of my own tears.

There's a saying, "salt water (sweat, tears, and the sea) wash away all ails." Energetically people are drawn to the ocean for vacations to wash away the worries, anxieties and stresses of their worlds. At the same time, a *good cry* and a *good sweat* are also both very healing. Chemically, sweat and tears both contain stress hormones, thus to cry and to sweat is your body's way of expelling, getting rid of, stress and restoring your body to baseline peace and calm.

I really learned the value of swimming in my own tears and moving them through my body in the early months of my divorce in 2013.

Separation from my husband of ten years was sudden and traumatic. He violently kicked me out of his life to become a monk. I detail the story and process of my healing in my memoir *The Gift Inside the Wound*. During that six months while I was homeless, lost, and broken, I experienced intense episodes of anxiety, panic, and worry like I never had before in my life. My personal practice during that time slowed down significantly. I often found myself spending most of the practice in Child's Pose, and moving more mindfully through sun salutations. That mindful approach revealed to me a whole new understanding of the power of water and flow in my body.

When I start flowing through some version of sun salutations, my tears almost always subside by the second or third salutation, and I feel my body moving the waters in my system. This flushes my bloodstream with the more calming hormones, pushing more stress hormones out, this time through my sweat. After several sun salutations, I feel myself letting go of whatever it was that made me cry, and able to move on to whatever is next.

By moving my body like water through sun salutations, I literally swam through my emotions. I allowed myself to fully *feel* the pains through my tears and push them out through my sweat. First I surrendered to my pain, then I moved it through and pushed it out, and finally I was able to step into the power of what is next.

Water is symbolic of the constant ebb and flow of changing moods and the tides of life. The world is always changing, ebbing, flowing, moving, and evolving. We cannot control what happens around us, nor can we control the madnesses that emerge from other people and circumstances. What we can control, is how we choose to engage with that ever-rotating, constantly churning, systematically spiraling world. When we choose to control how we respond, we learn to control our hormones. Water helps us to recognize that we aren't *supposed* to be anything, but rather we get to just *play* in the eddies and currents of life.

The point is, after swimming in one's own tears, you finally SURRENDER to who you are, as you are, and accept yourself as is. For me, linking my breath to the movements of sun-salutations always helps me find that letting-go and go-with-the-flow.

Every day during my divorce, as I practiced on my mat by myself, by the time I finished sun salutations, I was able to stop crying, pick myself up, and start to wonder with some level of curiosity what my life might be like post-divorce. Similarly, by the end of the chapter, Alice surrenders to the absurdity of Wonderland. She stops questioning the oddities around her and wishing for circumstances to be different. Rather, she accepts the weirdness of the world as it is, and she begins to converse with a mouse, a duck, a dodo, a lory, and an eaglet, who have also fallen into the pool with her. She recognizes that she is not alone in her pain, that those around her are swimming in the same kinds of emotions. Instead of fighting the strangeness of Wonderland, she goes with the flow of it and decides to contribute to the story.

5-Minute Practice
Half Sun Salutations

I GO WITH THE FLOW.
When I move with breath, I can FEEL to HEAL.
My emotions move through me.

Mountain Pose

Chair Pose

Half-Lift Pose

Ragdoll Pose

Half Lift Pose

Chair Pose

Mountain Pose

Sun Salutations A
Cheat Sheet

Tadasana

Utthitta Tadasana

Uttanasana

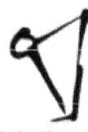

Ardha Uttanasana

Chaturanga Dandasana

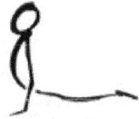

Urdhva Mukha Svanasana

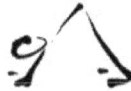

Adho Mukha Svanasana

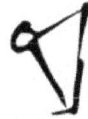

Ardha Uttanasana

Uttanasana

Utthitta Tadasana

Tadasana

Sun Salutations B
Cheat Sheet

Tadasana

Utkatasana

Uttanasana

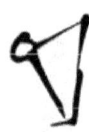

Ardha Uttanasana

Chaturanga Dandasana

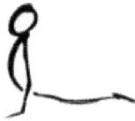

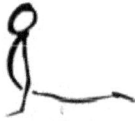

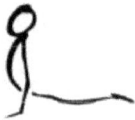

Urdhva Mukha Svanasana

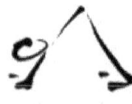

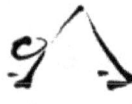

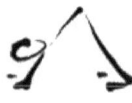

Adho Mukha Svanasana

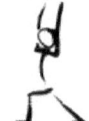

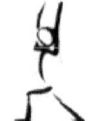

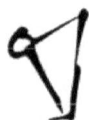

Virabhadrasana I

Chaturanga Dandasana

Urdhva Mukha Svanasana

Adho Mukha Svanasana

Virabhadrasana I

Chaturanga Dandasana

Urdhva Mukha Svanasana

Adho Mukha Svanasana

Ardha Uttanasana

Uttanasana

Utkatasana

Tadasana

Sun Salutations C
Cheat Sheet

Tadasana

Utthitta Tadasana

Uttanasana

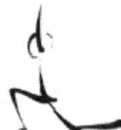

Anjaneyasana

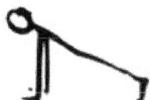

Plank

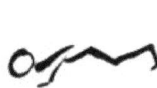

Ashtangasana

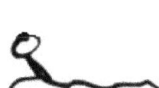

Bhujangasana

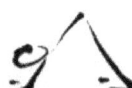

Adho Mukha Svanasana

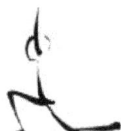

Anjaneyasana

Uttanasana

Utthitta Tadasana

Tadasana

Sun Salutations

ASANA

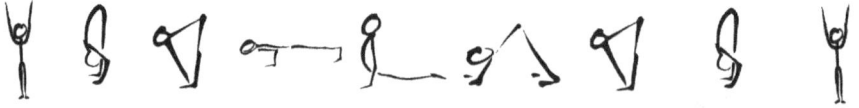

INTENTION

When I link my breath to my movement, I energize my life-force.
I honor and shine the light inside myself.
I move with intention.
I salute the light in myself and others.

Mountain

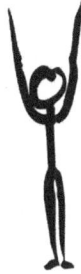

ASANA

INTENTION

> I can climb mountains and reach my summit.
> I am rooted, and tall.
> I am majestic, vast, powerful, and strong.
> I express the deepest wisdoms of my bones.

Chair Pose

ASANA

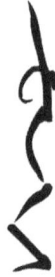

INTENTION

I take my seat at any table.
I am committed to my decisions and actions.
I am as fierce, powerful and strong as a thunderbolt.

Half-Lift

ASANA

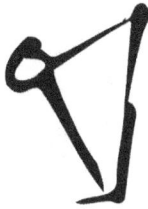

INTENTION

I find comfort in the space between places.
My length combined with my strength provides stability.
I turn inwards to express outwards.

Forward Fold (Ragdoll)

ASANA

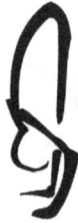

INTENTION

I can release and surrender, even in the midst of efforts.
I bow to the divine in myself.
I embody the balance of heaven and earth.

High-Low Plank

ASANA

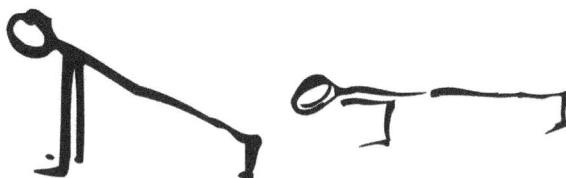

INTENTION

I am as solid, stable, and strong as an army.
I have the wisdom and comfort of a staff.
I am STABLE.

Inch Worm

ASANA

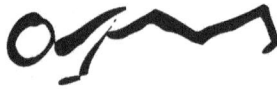

INTENTION

I can take things in tiny bite-sized steps.
Slow and steady wins the race.
Inch by inch, step by step.

Upward Dog

ASANA

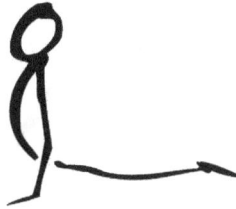

INTENTION

I am loyal and dedicated to my cause.
I am open and giving, while making space for my own needs.
I look forward while being planted in the NOW.

Downward Dog

ASANA

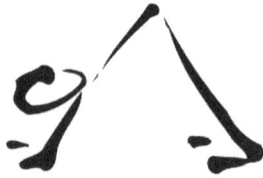

INTENTION

I am playful.
I play my part in cooperation.
I am comfortable in vulnerability.
I am loving and devoted.

Off the Mat Trick
MOZI Method to Go With the Flow

How to Let Go of Control and Wash Away Toxicity

Benefits
> ASANA - often tight low back and shoulder muscles will relax
> INTENTION - over-thinking, worry, anxiety & control will all decrease
> SPIRIT - you will feel more flexible and free

ASANA - MOVE
- Stand with feet hip-width apart and straight like #1s.
- Soften your knees
- Swivel your hips from side-to-side (like doing the twist)
- Shake your body

INTENTION - THINK
- "I go with the flow."
- "I let go of what is already out of my control."
- "I am flexible and free."
- "I shake it off."

SPIRIT - BREATHE
Breathe in as you stand still, breathe out as your swivel, shake, or dance.

Dosage
Practice this for 20-50 breaths a day, both when you need it and when you don't.
- 10 breaths when you wake up
- 3 breaths every time you wash you hands or are around water
- 5 breaths anytime you catch yourself holding on to control
- 10 breaths before getting into bed

Sun Salutations
Journal

Date/Time:

Mood

      Body -

      Mind -

      Spirit -

Intention

Practice Summary

Insight

The Dodo

Warrior Strength & Confidence
Warriors & Lunges

The Caucus Race - Everybody Wins

They were indeed a queer-looking party that assembled on the bank—the birds with draggled feathers, the animals with their fur clinging close to them, and all dripping wet, cross, and uncomfortable.

In Chapter III of *Alice's Adventures in Wonderland*, Alice and a variety of creatures arrive on the shore of a pool of Alice's tears, all looking like they have been through a terrible storm. The way these creatures are described as draggled feathers and fur clinging is exactly how I feel after many of the good hard cries I have had during sun salutations portion of my practice.

When I'm going through something rough in life, I often find myself a washed up mess of sweat, tears, and snot after sun sals, and ready to step into a different form of my strength.

The first question of course was, how to get dry again: they had a consultation about this, and after a few minutes it seemed quite natural to Alice to find herself talking familiarly with them.

At this point the Lory and the Mouse launch into discussion of things that they knew to be dry, namely a boring, inaccurate, and confused history lesson about William the Conquerer. Like the washed up creatures coming off the shore of the pool of tears, if I allow myself get too lost in the thoughts of my brain, I get confused and more distraught. How to get dry and move forward in my practice, my day, and my life can't happen by thinking and analyzing and trying to understand. The way to move forward isn't about analyzing the history (William the Conquerer), but rather in DOing something, actually taking action and moving forward.

Finally, the Dodo interrupts the dialogue and suggests a Caucus Race.

"In that case," said the Dodo solemnly, rising to its feet, "I move that the meeting adjourn, for the immediate adoption of more energetic remedies—. . .the best thing to get us dry would be a Caucus-race."

The Dodo's name says it all DO - DO! His suggestion is to stop thinking and discussing and DO!

When I finish sun salutations, the next step is to actually take a physical STEP, to put one foot forward and step into lunges and warriors and DO SOMETHING. The standing warrior poses are where action is taken, stepping forward and moving into new territory happens. In essence, the Dodo's suggestion to run a Caucus-race is to take a step in moving somewhere, AND to own your power as any candidate would do in a political caucus race.

There was no "One, two, three, and away," but they began running, when they liked, and left off when they liked, so that it was not easy to know when the race was over. However, when they had been running half-an hour or so, and were quite dry again, the Dodo suddenly called out, "The race is over!" and they all crowded round it, panting, and asking "But who has won?"

Like the Caucus- Race, life doesn't offer any rulebook, manual, or step-by-step process of order. As a result, people each take their own paths, scurrying about in a frenzy of doing this and doing that in their own way. On the spiritual path of stepping into new territory (as one does in warrior poses) everyone ends up having had similar experiences, gaining similar insights, and learning similar lessons, but they reach those lessons in their own way. In the same way, all the creatures run about in their own way, and ultimately they all get dry. In life, everyone is a spiritual warrior, taking his or her own course for the purpose of having a meaningful experience on this Earth.

At last the Dodo said, "Everybody has won, and all must have prizes."

Everybody wins, and receives a prize from the stash of treats and tidbits in Alice's pockets. Alice and the animals started the Caucus-Race without really knowing what it was they were doing except that they wanted to get dry (move on) from the wetness of the pool of tears. Whenever I step into warrior and lunge poses (without a teacher telling me what I'm doing or where I'm going) I am forced to have faith in myself, to run for myself and see what happens. I am a spiritual warrior stepping into the unknown with the faith that every experience will provide a valuable lesson. In the end, everybody wins.

5-Minute Practice Overview
Warriors & Lunges

I GO WITH THE FLOW.
When I move with breath, I can FEEL to HEAL.
My emotions move through me.

Runner's Lunge

Crescent Lunge

Humble Warrior

Warrior One

Warrior Two

Reverse Warrior

Runner's Lunge

ASANA

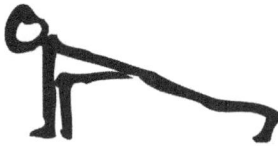

INTENTION

I trust in Spirit to lead me.
I am grounded in all steps I take in life.
I am supported in the present moment.
I acknowledge my past and look forward to my future.
I am long and strong.
I fully surrender to the Spirit and power within myself.
I trust Spirit to lead me.

Crescent Lunge

ASANA

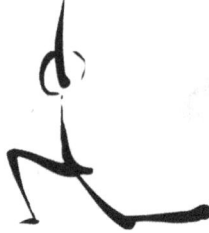

INTENTION

I grow up from the soil of my experiences.
I evolve to my fullest at my own pace.
I always have choice in my life.
I express the fullness of my being into the world
All things in my life come full circle.

Humble Warrior

ASANA

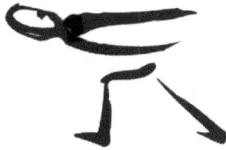

INTENTION

I bow to the Divine of Earth, and inside myself.
With my hands bound, I move forward from my heart.
I surrender, guided by Spirit, in every step I take.
I am humble.
I greet everyone in humility, honesty, and authenticity.

Warrior I

ASANA

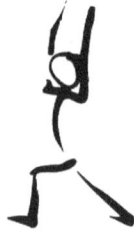

INTENTION

I am prepared to step into the unknown.
I am mindful of every step I take.
My past experiences prepared me for future steps
I am open-minded and receptive to the wisdom of Spirit.
I am humble.

Warrior 2

ASANA

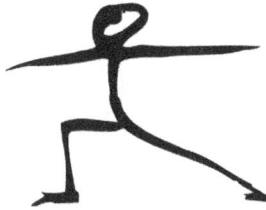

INTENTION

My past experience have prepared me to step into the unknown.
I am grounded and stable as I step into new directions.
I step into new experience with confidence & stability.
I maintain the courage of a spiritual warrior.
I am a spiritual warrior.
I am equally open to giving and receiving.
I have the strength in me to do and go anywhere.

Reverse Warrior

ASANA

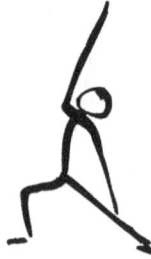

INTENTION

I release attachments to results as I step forward with confidence.
I remain solid in the present moment as I reach upwards.
I am awakened and invigorated
I create space and openness to receive gifts from my efforts.
I am open to receive abundance from the Universe.

Off the Mat Trick
MOZI Method Access Your Strength

How to Feel Confident & Self- Assured

Benefits

ASANA -increased strength & endurance

INTENTION - increased confidence & sense of self-worth

SPIRIT - you will feel empowered and invincible

ASANA - MOVE

- Stand with feet hip-width apart and straight like #1s.
- Soften your knees
- Align your ribs over your hips
- Gently hug/embrace your belly

INTENTION - THINK

- "I and strong and powerful."
- "I believe in myself and my purpose."
- "I am confident and competent"
- "I've got this!"

SPIRIT - BREATHE

Breathe in as you stand still, breathe out as you hug your belly and exert strength.

Dosage

Practice this for 20-50 breaths a day, both when you need it and when you don't.

- 10 breaths when you wake up
- 3 breaths every time you look in a mirror
- 5 breaths anytime you exert effort or need strength
- 10 breaths before getting into bed

Warriors & Lunges
Journal

Date/Time:

Mood

      Body -

      Mind -

      Spirit -

Intention

Practice Summary

Insight

The Mouse's Long Tale

Twist into Center
Standing Twist Poses

It is a Long Tail

"It is a long tail, certainly," said Alice, looking down with wonder at the Mouse's tail; "but why do you call it sad?" And she kept on puzzling about it while the Mouse was speaking,

In Chapter III of *Alice's Adventures in Wonderland*, Alice asks a mouse to explain why it doesn't like cats or dogs. The mouse's tale, like its tail, twists and turns many times, and Alice cannot keep up with the story. The mouse's sad tale, which is written in the shape of a tail down the page, describes someone being on trial with a judge and jury condemning them to death.

The mouse's tale/tail exemplifies how life can take many unfair twists and turns, and if we aren't careful, we can turn in on ourselves and twist into a knot. I've found that especially after I've been through a harrowing "warrior" type experience in my life, I can get too caught up in the twists and turns of the world around me. This leads to me losing focus of where I want to go in the first place. While I try to remind myself that the twists and turns and blocks and challenges along my path ARE my path, I sometimes do feel like I'm turning myself into a knot. Doing twist poses, reminds me to stop looking at the twists and turns in the outside world, but rather to twist in on myself, to look inside myself..

For Alice and the Mouse, Fury is name of the dog that causes so much turmoil. Perhaps Lewis Carroll named the dog Fury in reference to the three Greek Goddesses called the *Furies*. In Greek mythology, a *Fury* is described as an angry fire that pursues and punishes wrong-doers.

"You are not attending!" said the Mouse to Alice severely. "What are you thinking of?"

"I beg your pardon," said Alice very humbly: "you had got to the fifth bend, I think?"

"I had not!" cried the Mouse, sharply and very angrily.

The further the Mouse twists in on his tale/tail, the more passion anger he builds, and eventually he spits his fire out on Alice, accusing her of not paying close enough attention.

After years of teaching yoga classes, I've come to realize that yoga practitioners commonly feel angry during twisting poses, as they release old patterns and emotions. To me, it is no coincidence that twist poses activate an internal fire in my belly, a radiating heat that erupts out of me (like a *fury*) that ignites a passion (or rage) in my energy. One of the purposes of yoga is to remind you to spiral into yourself, to find the fire and passion within you, to connect with Spirit within you. Twisting poses physically put you in a position to spiral into your center, to go deeper and deeper into yourself, and find the core where *Fury* resides.

> an old crab took the opportunity of saying to her daughter, "Ah, my dear! Let this be a lesson to you never to lose your temper!"

> "Hold your tongue, Ma!" said the young crab, a little snappishly, "You're enough to try the patience of an oyster!"

One of the most difficult lessons of life, in my experience, is the lesson of balancing the thin line between passion and anger. I always say to my clients that I like anger, because it means action. When we feel anger, we get a surge of adrenaline and other stress hormones that push us to action to *change* something. Yet, we must be careful to not spit our anger and fire at others, but rather to use it to inspire and motivate others through our passion. As the crab says, we must not lose our temper, but rather control it.

> "I wish I had our Dinah here, I know I do!" said Alice aloud, addressing nobody in particular. "She'd soon fetch it back!"

> "And who is Dinah, if I might venture to ask the question?" said the Lory.

Alice replied eagerly, for she was always ready to talk about her pet. "Dinah's our cat. And she's such a capital one for catching mice, you can't think! And oh, I wish you could see her after the birds! Why, she'll eat a little bird as soon as look at it!"...

On various pretexts they all moved off, and Alice was soon left alone.

Alice expressed her own passion, about her cat Dinah, but her passion was too hot and scary for the creatures of Wonderland. They were scared off by the talk of the cat and soon left Alice all alone, leaving her to contemplate how her own *fury* scared away her companions.

Twisting poses are a practice in accessing your *fury*, your internal fire, and keeping that fire in just the right control so as to use it for passion and drive rather than anger and rage. The spiral represents centeredness, the radiation of energy, the expansion of Self, evolution, and the awareness of the unity of all things. When you spiral in on yourself with control, you access your core authenticity and radiate it out to the world. The spiral is one of the world's oldest symbols, revealing itself in the double helix of DNA, the swirling action of the Milky Way galaxy, seashells, and animal horns.

Alice's adventures in Wonderland are a journey for her to find her true self and learn how to express herself to the outside world, no matter how foreign that world may be. The Mouse's long tale/tail is part of her process in turning in on herself and what is passionate to her, while finding healthy ways to express that out to others in a way that they will receive her. Twisting poses support this turning inward process.

5-Minute Practice Overview
Standing Twists

I turn inward to myself.
I know what is right for me at my core.
I turn inward to express outward.

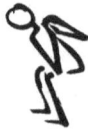 Chair Twist

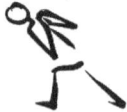 Lunge Twist

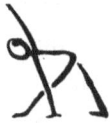 Twisting Triangle

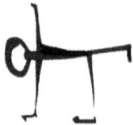 Twisting Half-Moon

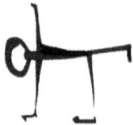 Squat Twist

Chair Twist

ASANA

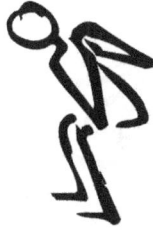

INTENTION

I am stable, no matter what swirls around me.
From my base to my crown, I am centered.
My heart leads all my actions and motions.
I am compassionate, open, and loving.

Lunge Twist

ASANA

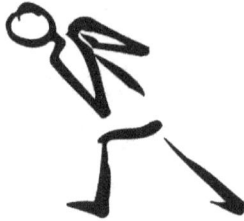

INTENTION

I am calm in the midst of fire.
I am centered, no matter what.
I am safe to let go of whatever no longer serves me.
I release my intense emotions.
I breathe freely, in and out, giving and receiving, through turmoil.
I am able to process and digest any circumstance.

Twisting Triangle

ASANA

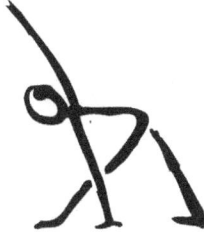

INTENTION

I am stable, balanced & safe in the midst of confusion.
I am centered, no matter what.
I create space and openness in my life.
I can view experiences from many perspectives.
I take in life fully in every situation and challenge.

Twisting Half-Moon

ASANA

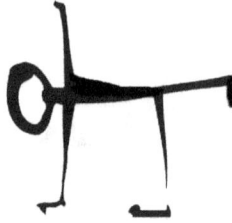

INTENTION

I am solid, grounded, and stable, even when off balance.
I anchor in the earth below to grasp Heaven around me.
I am supported by my own strength.
I am centered.
I am strong & independent.
I stand true in my Self in all I do.
Even while challenged, I express compassion & love.
My focus guides my purpose & intention.

Squat Twist (Noose)

ASANA

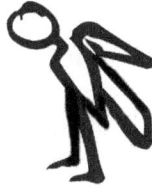

INTENTION

I am brought closer to Mother Earth, supported & stable.
Whatever no longer serves me is pushed out.
I hug and love myself, exactly as I am.
I "noose" my ego to access humility.
I feel and act from love and compassion.

Off the Mat Trick
MOZI Method – Turn Within

Benefits

ASANA -increased core strength & flexibility

INTENTION - improved confidence & self-worth

SPIRIT - you will feel able to step outside your comfort zone

ASANA - MOVE

- Align your ribs over your hips
- Softly engage belly muscles (uddi)
- Hug yourself, right hand on left ribs, left hand on right ribs
- Slowly twist your ribs from side to side with your breath

INTENTION - THINK

- "I turn within myself."
- "I know myself at my core."
- "I stay true to my core"
- "I express myself outwardly"

SPIRIT - BREATHE

Breathe in as your twist one way, breathe out as you twist the other way.

Dosage

Practice this for 20-50 breaths a day, both when you need it and when you don't.

- 10 breaths when you wake up
- 3 breaths every time you look in a mirror
- 5 breaths when you need to step outside your comfort zone
- 10 breaths before getting into bed

Standing Twists
Journal

Date/Time:

Mood

      Body -

      Mind -

      Spirit -

Intention

Practice Summary

Insight

In a Little Bill

Losing & Re-Gaining Balance
Standing Balance Poses

Everything is Changed

It was the White Rabbit, trotting slowly back again, and looking anxiously about as it went, as if it had lost something; and she heard it muttering to itself, "The Duchess! The Duchess! O my dear paws! Oh my fire and whiskers! She'll get me executed, as sure as ferrets are ferrets! Where can I have dropped them, I wonder!"

—everything seemed to have changed since her swim in the pool, and the great hall, with the glass table and the little door, had vanished completely.

In Chapter IV of *Alice's Adventures in Wonderland,* Alice encounters the White Rabbit, quite distraught as he has lost his fan and white gloves. Without his tools, the White Rabbit appears off his center, and Alice sees that the White Rabbit has flaws like anyone else. She can no longer look to him to lead her, but rather, must figure out how to balance on her own feet and find her own way.

As I have alluded to the White Rabbits of yoga as our yoga instructors, there comes a time in every student/teacher relationship, where the student recognizes that the teacher has flaws. While we may still want to look at our teachers to lead us, the truth is that the answers lie within ourselves, and we must find our own way to stand on our own two feet. The standing balance series is symbolic of losing our ground and having to regain balance when a leg (our White Rabbit) is taken from us.

"Why Mary Ann, what are you doing out here? Run home this moment, and fetch me a pair of gloves and a fan! Quick now!" And Alice was so much frightened that she ran off at once in the direction it pointed to. . .

"He took me for his housemaid," she said to herself as she ran. "How surprised he'll be when he finds out who I am!"

While Alice agrees to help the White Rabbit, at the same time, she asserts to herself that *she knows who she is!*   Her identity crisis of growing and shrinking and not knowing how she belongs in this foreign world has passed. Alice has gained a sense of confidence in her adventures that she didn't have before, and now she is seeing the White Rabbit in a moment of weakness.

In yoga, that point where the student recognizes the humanity and flaws and foibles of the teacher, the student is faced with the reality of walking on their own, without their teacher. In some cases, this happens community-wide. For example, in 2012 John Friend, founder of Anusara Yoga, came tumbling off his pedestal when several of his staff accused him of embezzlement, sexual harassment and other unethical behaviors. From 2014-2016, Bikram Choudhury, founder of Bikram Yoga and the father of the Hot Yoga movement faced several lawsuits of fraud and harassment. He eventually fled the country.

As a small local teacher, I was not immune to the teacher/student disillusionment factor either. I opened small yoga studio in 2005, which I closed and filed bankruptcy just two years later. My students were devastated, and at the same time, they saw my humanity and my flaws. Many of them told me after my studio closed that they felt like they had lost a leg, their stability, that they had to figure out how to stand for themselves.

I have since come to believe that the White Rabbits of life, our teachers and guides and gurus, always come tumbling down off the pedestals on which we place them. Thus, in my own approach to teaching, I now choose to step down myself. When I see that a student no longer needs me to give them guidance, I encourage them to move on without me. While I tell them I will always be there to encourage and affirm them, I give them my *graduation talk*. I tell them they no longer need me to tell them what to do or how to do it. I tell them that they are always welcome to come back and visit me, and even seek me out to offer the encouragement and affirmation but that they no longer need me to be their teacher.

her eye fell upon a little bottle that stood near the looking-glass. There was no label this time with the words "DRINK ME," but nevertheless she uncorked it and put it to her lips.

After seeing the White Rabbit in his weakness, Alice chooses to drink another potion, this time without any authority (the DRINK ME tag) telling her to do so. Instead, she makes the choice on her own. In doing so, she crosses a threshold, a point of no return, where she completely surrenders to the happenings of Wonderland, with confidence in her ability to handle whatever may happen.

Whenever I give a student the *graduation talk,* they usually get mad at me as they all go through a sort of unsteadiness on their feet (like balance poses) because they have to figure out how to balance themselves without me showing them how. Just like the communities of Bikram and Anusara had to figure out a new way, my students have to find their own legs. It's a "point of no return" when the teacher leaves the student and the student must find a way to balance on their own, without a teacher to lean on. The student has to graduate, to grow up.

I'm grown up now," she added in a sorrowful tone, "at least there's no room to grow up any more here." . . .

she was now about a thousand times as large as the Rabbit, and had no reason to be afraid of it.

When the potion finally takes its full effect and Alice stops growing, she ends up with her foot up the chimney, her arm out the window, and no way to move, much less get out of the house. She has a conversation with herself, a back and forth (balancing both sides) conversation with HERSELF.

"Oh, you foolish Alice!" she answered herself. "How can you learn lessons in here? Why, there's hardly room for you, and no room at all for any lesson-books!"

When left alone, without a teacher, we may feel limited, awkward in our own bodies. We cannot rely on lesson-books and teachers anymore. Standing balance poses reveal to use the tiniest of imbalances in our systems, and we may feel off balance, over tight, unable to move as we would like (like Alice trapped in the house). Yet, we practice balance. We go back and forth, side to side, in standing balances, as if having a back-and-forth conversation with ourselves through our own bodies.

"We must burn the house down!" said the Rabbit's voice, and Alice called out as loud as she could, "if you do, I'll set Dinah at you!"

Alice listens as the White Rabbit works in concert with several other creatures to try to free her from the house. At this point, Alice is no longer afraid of, nor submissive to the White Rabbit. Rather, she takes authority over herself and even resists the help being offered. First she swats at the White Rabbit at the window; then she kicks Little Bill, a lizard, out of the chimney, and finally she threatens them with her cat (because she knows they are all terrified of Dinah the cat). She became the authority, even though it became clear that the White Rabbit held a high position as the community judge.

Like Alice, once I trusted myself to be "grown up" in my practice, I rejected the support of teachers for a time. When I did try to take classes, I was resistant, reluctant, and even recalcitrant in receiving suggestions from the teachers leading the class. I'd put myself in the back row, tell them that I go at my own pace, and skip poses that didn't feel right to me, or scoff in my mind at sequences I thought were unreasonable or unhealthy. I became every yoga teacher's worst nightmare.

Yoga teachers all know these students, the know-it-alls who do their own thing and refuse to listen to instruction. It's part of the yoga growth process. Like Alice swatting at the Rabbit out the window and kicking Little Bill out of the chimney, we have to reject the teacher in order to find our own authority.

And yet, in my cockiness, I lost the power of humility. Thankfully, the power of being humble was always brought back to me in standing balance poses, where I would *always* fall if I got too arrogant. Like Alice, in rejecting the suggestions of teachers and getting too cocky about it, I also found myself *stuck* in a position that dis-allowed anymore growth. I had to shrink back down to size.

a shower of little pebbles came rattling in at the window, and some of them hit her in the face. . . Alice noticed with some surprise that the pebbles were all turning into little cakes as they lay on the floor. . . So she swallowed one of the cakes, and was delighted to find that she began shrinking directly.

Alice does need the help of the White Rabbit, as she needs the pebbles turned to cakes to shrink her back to size. However, the creatures do not tell her what the pebbles are for when they toss them to her. They cannot force her to eat them once they turn to cakes anymore than they can tell her how many to eat to get to the right size. She must figure out all these things on her own. She must hold her own authority, and yet learn how to be humble enough to work together with others in a challenge.

Like Alice, in my home practice, I needed to learn how to listen and take in the advice of others, reject what didn't feel right (kick Little Bill out of the chimney) and accept what did feel right (eat the cakes).

5-Minute Practice Overview
Standing Balance

I balance all options and know what is right for ME.
I am balanced and stable in myself.
I am a balance of confident and humble.

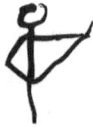 Eagle

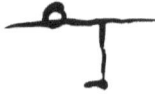 Leg Raise

Warrior Three

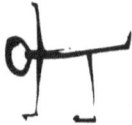 Half-Moon

Tree

Eagle Pose

ASANA

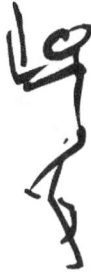

INTENTION

I am connected to my humanity as I tap into the energy of greatness.
I am large and humble.
I am centered and balanced.
My masculine and feminine aspects merge.
Even with wings clipped, I access the energy of my heart.
Through compression I achieve expression
I have keen vision, seeing my circumstances and environment
clearly.

Leg Raise (front & side)

ASANA

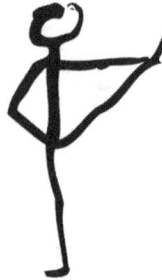

INTENTION

I am balanced even when supported by only half my foundation.
Grace is always available to me.
I stand tall through whatever comes my way.
I always return home to my own heart.
I stay strong even when taking unfamiliar and awkward actions.

Warrior Three

ASANA

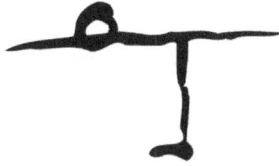

INTENTION

I am grounded as I launch into new directions.
I am always connected to the strength and power within me.
My love and passion reach out from my heart center.
I see the vast possibilities.
I commit to the spiritual journey that is offered me.
I am balanced between my past and my future, in this moment.
I am grounded as I fly.
I am anchored in my center, radiating outward.

Half Moon

ASANA

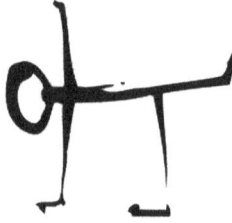

INTENTION

I am supported as I open to full exposure.
I draw strength from the earth below as I give myself in service.
I tap into the playful child inside me.
I am open, compassionate, and loving.
I am balanced.
I play BIG!

Tree

ASANA

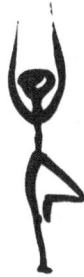

INTENTION

I root down to rise up.
I am nourished, supported, and anchored.
I am giving and opening of myself to others in my grove.
I am love.
I express love.
I grow with love.
I am wise.
Like a tree, I am connected to everything on earth.
As above, so below, through me.

Off the Mat Trick
MOZI Method – Balance

Benefits

ASANA -increased balance & stability

INTENTION - improved adaptability and playfulness

SPIRIT - you will find fun in failure

ASANA - MOVE

- Stand in mountain pose, even on both feet
- Lift one foot, and purposely shift your weight until you lose your balance
- Watch and feel yourself catch your balance

INTENTION - THINK

- "I adapt to anything and everything that happens"
- "I play BIG."
- "I catch myself when I fall"
- "Falling is learning, and fun"

SPIRIT - BREATHE

Breathe in as root down, breathe out as you allow yourself to fall. Breathe in as you come back to balanced center.

Dosage

Practice this for 20-50 breaths a day, both when you need it and when you don't.

- 10 breaths when you wake up
- while waiting (I do it while waiting for my dog to pee on a walk)
- 5 breaths when you get bored and need some fun
- 10 breaths before getting into bed

Standing Balance
Journal

Date/Time:

Mood

> Body -
>
> Mind -
>
> Spirit -

Intention

Practice Summary

Insight

Advice from a Caterpillar

Transition & Transformation
Standing Angle Poses

Changed Several Times

"Who are you?" said the Caterpillar.
This was not an encouraging opening for a conversation.
Alice replied, rather shyly, "I-I hardly know, sir, just at
present—at least I know who I was when I got up this
morning, but I think I must have been changed several
times since then."

In Chapter V of *Alice's Adventures in Wonderland,* Alice encounters a hookah smoking caterpillar sitting atop a mushroom. In conversation with the caterpillar, Alice implies that she knew who she was before entering Wonderland, but so many things have changed since then that she doesn't recognize herself anymore (specifically she has grown and shrunk to many different physical sizes).

Yoga practitioners, especially those who have gone through yoga teacher training, can relate to Alice at this point. Those who have committed to a serious practice know that it changes you, deeply. And continues to change you, over and over and over again. A consistent practice changes so many things about your body, your perspective, your behavior, and how you engage in your life, and change continues over time.

For me, the changes were both subtle and drastic. Within the first year of taking yoga seriously, I quit my job, moved to a different state, got engaged and married, and started teaching yoga. I was also hit by a truck as a pedestrian, and somehow healed from those injuries and straightened a lifelong scoliosis at the same time. Yoga made me into a whole new person, and in many ways, I didn't recognize myself as I once used to be.

"being so many different sizes in a day is very confusing."

"It isn't," said the Caterpillar.

"Well, perhaps you haven't found it so yet," said Alice;
"but when you have to turn into a chrysalis—you will
some day, you know—and then after that into a

butterfly, I should think you'll feel it a little queer, won't you?"

"Not a bit," said the Caterpillar

While Alice laments that all the changes are rather confusing, the caterpillar contradicts her by simply saying that it isn't. From the perspective of a caterpillar, change is a necessary and ordinary and beautiful part of the process of life. In fact, for a caterpillar, changing from a caterpillar to a chrysalis to a butterfly is not only natural, but expected. Perhaps the caterpillar is there to urge Alice to surrender to the changes and accept that transition, transformation and change are all beautiful parts of the process of life.

For me, some of the changes I experienced were really fun, like getting married, and others were really difficult, like getting a new job and realizing that I no longer enjoyed my industry. Sometimes the changes took longer to evolve, and other ones were rather sudden. But what I did realize rather quickly was that after starting yoga, my life wasn't as mundane or consistent anymore. Everything was changing all the time. Big things. I couldn't fight it. Rather, I had to surrender to it. I had to look at it like an adventure rather than a challenge.

One of the greatest teachings in yoga (and many other spiritual traditions) is that the only true constant in life is change. There's a saying in Maui, Hawaii. *If you don't like the weather, wait five minutes.* This adage reminds people that everything changes, eventually. Some things more slowly than others, but the ultimate truth is change is inevitable, eventually. In yoga, you don't spend eternity in one pose. It eventually changes. And in some traditions (hot yoga) the teacher even emphasizes the word *CHANGE* as the cue to transition or transform. Thus, the practice of yoga is about taking the changing processes of life with ease and grace and beauty, just as a caterpillar does when it changes to a chrysalis and then into a butterfly.

For some minutes, it puffed away without speaking, but at last it unfolded its arms, took the hookah out of its mouth again, and said, "So you think you're changed, do you?"

The caterpillar is a sage figure who speaks in calm tones with long gaps of silence. He takes his time to contemplate his thoughts before speaking, and when he does, he challenges Alice to step outside her paradigm into a new kind of thinking. In this passage, he suggests that even though she has changed sizes time and again, he asks her to consider if she has *really* changed, what she *really* wants to be, what contentment means to her, and finally suggests that she will eventually get used to all the changes.

> . . ."What size do you want to be?". . .Are you content now?". . .

Throughout their conversation, the caterpillar poses many questions to Alice, urging her to contemplate her circumstance without ever really giving her any direct advice. His steady voice is symbolic of the still, small voice of intuition that yoga practitioners seek to hear in themselves. Like the caterpillar, our intuition often contradicts logic, and challenges us to contemplate *really* what we think and want to do. Yet it is the one *true* voice that is always right.

From a spiritual perspective of yoga, the caterpillar has an interesting point to ponder. While yes, our worlds and how we react in our worlds can change drastically, and everything does in fact change, at the core of our essence, we do essentially stay the same. In essence, the caterpillar challenges Alice to surrender to the constant state of change, and at the same time recognize that still small steadiness inside herself that doesn't change, her Truth.

After about a decade of yoga practice, having completed several of my own trainings, teaching for several years, and leading several teacher trainings, I came to a pretty revolutionary realization. I was revising curriculum for my next yoga teacher training, writing it out in detailed lesson plans so that I could mentor other trainers to run it when I recognized that I was a TEACHER. I had gone to college and grad school to teach, and even though I had long since given up my K-12 certification, I was still teaching. While many things on the outside (zip code, marital status, tax filing forms) had changed, one thing hadn't changed, my love of teaching and writing. At my core, I was always the same.

"But I'm not used to it!" pleaded poor Alice in a piteous tone. And she thought to herself, "I wish the creatures wouldn't be so easily offended."

"You'll get used to it in time," said the Caterpillar; and it put the hookah into its mouth and began smoking again.

Alice wants to control the changes that are happening to her. In Wonderland, she experienced a complete paradigm shift. When she tried to apply what she knew and understood about life in her normal world to Wonderland, nothing made sense anymore. She could not expect everything to always stay the same, as much as she would like the constancy as stability. The caterpillar teaches Alice that transformation and change, especially in Wonderland, are inevitable, and uncontrollable. Yet, once she contemplates all his questions and finds patience and stillness (she waits patiently for him to speak again) he gives her the information she desires, how to control the growing and shrinking.

In my own experience, after over a decade of riding the roller coaster of significant life changes, the biggest one of all hit me. My husband left me to become a celibate monk. I found myself divorcing, homeless, and having to reinvent myself yet again. Like Alice, I didn't want the people around me to judge me, and I didn't think I would ever get used to the constant changing. I wished, like that caterpillar told Alice, that I would get used to it in time.

This time Alice waited patiently until it chose to speak again. In a minute or two the Caterpillar took the hookah out of its mouth and yawned once or twice, and shook itself. Then it got down off the mushroom, and crawled away into the grass, merely remarking as it went, "One side will make you grow taller, and the other side will make you grow shorter."

Similarly, yoga students eventually learn that the essence of yoga is adjusting to all kinds of internal and external circumstances while remaining centered and at peace within yourself. Yoga is centeredness, standing in your true nature, despite any outside forces, challenges, excuses, logic, reasons, or explanations.

At the same time, yoga students are often eager or anxious that yoga practice will help them achieve or attain a state of *enlightenment* or *realization*. My ex-husband was one who was always striving to reach enlightenment. He wanted the *liberation* that happened to many a spiritual guru.

But, like the caterpillar becoming a butterfly, transformation is not something that can be achieved, but something that occurs naturally over time. The caterpillar is neither anxious nor eager about the impending change of becoming a butterfly one day, and does not strive for transformation, it just happens as it is meant to occur. Enlightenment is not attained or achieved, but rather is a state that is eventually recognized or remembered as part of the natural order of the change process. It is through the surrendering to the process and journey of transition, not in striving for the end result of the transformation, that you remember the ultimate Truth.

5-Minute Practice Overview
Standing Angle Poses

I let go of the old in order to accept the new.
I allow myself to transition, transform and change.
Change is GOOD!

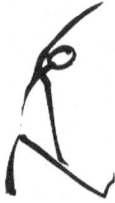 Gate Pose

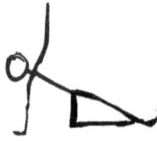 Side Plank

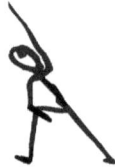 Side Angle Pose

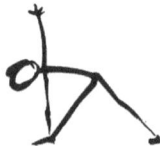 Triangle Pose

Gate Pose

ASANA

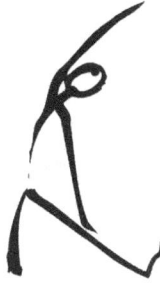

INTENTION

I am humble (on my knee) and open to guidance.
I awaken to the fullness of experience.
I am safe and supported by the ground beneath me.
My efforts are balanced and equal.
I maintain equilibrium over a large space.
I walk through the gateway with confidence.
I step through the portal from one space to another with grace.

Side Plank

ASANA

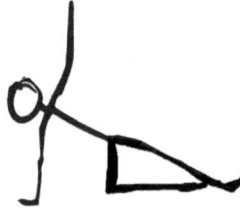

INTENTION

My arms serve as an extension of my heart.
I am balanced, solid, straight, and strong.
I am both large and humble.
I am connected to all things all directions.

Side Angle Pose

ASANA

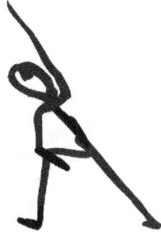

INTENTION

I am a warrior of stability.
I am a conduit of energy between spirit and earth.
I am firmly planted in my experience & open to possibilities.
I open and remove blocks to my potential.
My internal fire radiates through all my limbs in full expression.
I experience life beyond the limits of my body.

Triangle Pose

ASANA

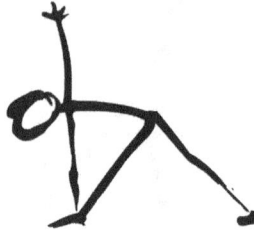

INTENTION

I am anchored by my past (back leg).
I am stable in my present (hips)
I am solid in my future (front leg).
My strength provides a sense of home wherever I am.
I am supported.
I am centered.
I grow and evolve in every direction and aspect of life.
What I let go creates space for something new.
My arms are an extension and expression of my heart.
I am able to see situations from a greater perspective.

Off the Mat Trick
MOZI Method - Transition

Benefits

ASANA -grounding & centeredness

INTENTION - calm through change

SPIRIT - you will find adventure in changes

ASANA - MOVE

- Walk SLOWLY
- Pause for a moment between steps, when both feet are grounded
- Pay attention as you transfer the weight from one foot to the other, and pause at that moment when the weight is equal in both feet

INTENTION - THINK

- "I stay calm through transition"
- "I adapt to change"
- "I transform with grace"
- "The only constant is change, and I adapt with ease"

SPIRIT - BREATHE

Breathe in as you step and shift your weight.

Breathe out as you pause with your weight even in both feet.

Dosage

Practice this for 20-50 breaths a day, both when you need it and when you don't.

- 10 steps while walking to the bathroom after waking up
- every time you walk to your car or bathroom
- 2 breaths as you walk through doorways
- 10 steps before getting into bed

Standing Angle Poses
Journal

Date/Time:

Mood

      Body -

      Mind -

      Spirit -

Intention

Practice Summary

Insight

The Cheshire Cat

Non-Attachment
Standing Forward Folds

It Doesn't Matter Which Way

"Would you tell me, please, which way I ought to walk from here?"
"That depends a good deal on where you want to get to," said the Cat.
"I don't much care where—" said Alice.
"Then it doesn't matter which way you walk," said the Cat.
"—so long as I get somewhere," Alice added as explanation.
"Oh, you're sure to do that," said the Cat,"if you only walk long enough."

In Chapter VI of *Alice's Adventures in Wonderland,* Alice encounters the Cheshire Cat, sitting on the branch of a tree. The cat is described as looking goodnatured, with very long claws and a great many teeth, leading Alice to believe she should treat it with respect. Their conversation, on the surface, looks to be a simple one of stating generalized facts. Alice asks for directions, the Cat asks her where she wants to go. However, at this point in her adventures, Alice has surrendered completely to the oddities of her experiences, and she has no preferences. She just wants to enjoy the experience.

One of the basic spiritual tenets of yoga is the concept of *aparigraha* or non-attachment. Another way to look at this *yama* (moral restraint) is to think of it as letting go of preferences and being open to possibilities. As Alice is surrendered to her adventures, she has no attachment to where she goes, and therefore she is open to the possibilities of the excitements of her adventures. The Cheshire Cat here represents the exuberant joy of non-attachment, and the thrill of the adventure that comes with being open to possibilities. The only preference Alice offers is that she would like to go *somewhere,* asserting what was learned in the prior chapter about transition and transformation. Alice, like yogis, has accepted the idea that the only constant is change, so she suggests that she might like to explore the fun that comes with transition, transformation, and change. Letting go is perhaps one of the most difficult spiritual lessons to embrace. We are psychologically conditioned as young children to develop preferences, to attach to desires, to set and reach for goals. The lesson of *aparigraha* is a practice in balancing the opposing energies of letting go of desires with holding on to intentions. Alice does this when she lets go of her specific desires of how she used to be, yet she hangs onto her general desire to have an adventure and go *somewhere*.

For me, when I finally surrendered to the fact that yoga was changing me, and accepted that in the big picture of it all, the changes were things I wanted (even though they were sometimes uncomfortable) I also surrendered my desires to hold on to things from my past. I let go of my identity as a public school teacher, a wife, a homeowner. In doing so, I also had to let go of knowing where I was going next. Like Alice, I knew I wanted to go *somewhere* and I knew that wherever *somewhere* was, it would bring with it an adventure. So, in the winter of 2013, I packed up my Prius and started on what turned out to be a five year adventure of homelessness. While I did have control of which way my car drove, I had no clue what adventures I would have in those places.

The same thing happens on my yoga mat every single day I practice without a teacher. I have control over the fact that I want to practice, and I want to do *something* on my mat. I even get to choose which poses I'm gonna practice each day. But I have absolutely no control over what I experience or learn in each practice. Therein lies the adventure.

> *"In that direction," the Cat said, waving its right paw round, "lives a Hatter: and in that direction," waving the other paw, "lives a March Hare. Visit either you like: they're both mad."*
> *"But I don't want to go among mad people," Alice remarked.*
> *"Oh, you can't help that," said the Cat: "we're all mad here. I'm mad. You're mad." . . .*
> *"How do you know I'm mad?" said Alice.*
> *"You must be," said the Cat, "or you wouldn't have come here."*

The Cheshire Cat offers some general insight as to what Alice will encounter in each of two different directions, and suggests to her that whichever path she takes, she will encounter madness. To take it a step further, the Cat suggests that Alice herself is mad. The two directions the Cheshire Cat suggests lead her to places of madness. But what exactly is *madness*? Did it mean the same thing to Lewis Carroll as he wrote about Alice in the mid 1800s as it does to us today? What does the word *madness* really mean?

The Mad Hatter is a reference to the 1829 phrase "mad as a hatter" which implies that hatter's went mad from prolonged exposure to the chemicals (mercurous nitrate) used in curing felt for hats. The March Hare is a reference to the phrase "mad as a March Hare" which originated in the 1500s alluding to the excitable and erratic behavior of hares in the breeding season, which occurs in March. Notably, however, the etymology of the word *madness* has connotations marking even further back to the 1400s indicating that madness is not just about about craziness or insanity, but rather also about being "beside oneself with excitement or enthusiasm, under the influence of uncontrollable emotion."

Perhaps prolonged exposure to the hormone and internal chemical changes that occur as a result of yoga practice produces a state of madness, not unlike (but also quite different from) that of a mad hatter. Perhaps the shifts in energies and endorphins that occur as a result of yoga practice is quite similar to the shifts in energies of breeding hares in the springtime. In many ways, the Cheshire Cat is correct. We are all mad. We all have chemical hormones in our systems, and they are subject to changes and adjustments and causing enthusiastic behaviors at any time. Anyone who has committed to a serious yoga practice can attest to the fact that it changes how you feel, and your world is quite different after yoga than it was before. And, it is my experience that people who don't practice yoga do, in some ways, look at yoga practitioners as if we are all mad.

When I left my entire world behind and set out to live out of my Prius, traveling from state to state to teach yoga wherever anyone would have me, for the pure adventure of it all, many people thought I was mad. And at the same time, many people were secretly envious of my courage. Everywhere I went, I carried my yoga mat. I rolled out my mat in hundreds of odd locations, with a sort of obsessed madness. No matter what, I practiced, a minimum of 20 minutes, five days a week. And always, after every single practice, I rolled my mat back up with a big toothy Cheshire grin on my face, like a happy cat who had just drunk a large saucer of fine cream. That grin always always lingers.

> *and this time [the Cat] vanished quite slowly, beginning with the end of the tail, and ending with the grin, which remained some time after the rest of it had gone.*

As the cat vanishes, leaving its grin to linger, it once again represents the concept of non-attachment, *aparigraha*. For Alice, this is yet another curious phenomenon of Wonderland. For yogis, it affirms that concept that non-attachment, letting go of desires in order to embrace possibilities will leave you with a lingering grin, an inner joy that lasts.

> *"Well! I've often seen a cat without a grin," thought Alice; "but a grin without a cat! It's the most curious thing I ever saw in all my life!"*

The more Alice surrenders to the madness and curiosity of Wonderland, the more she comes to expect the unexpected. Similarly, the more you learn to surrender in yoga practice—something you will particularly learn to do as you take standing forward folds—the more you will be able to handle the madness and chaos of the world off your mat.

Yoga instructors often speak of "'getting out of your head" or "dropping your thoughts"—not unlike the Red Queen's threats to "Chop off her head!," the first of many references to the beheading to come. (Later in the book, the Queen orders beheadings just about as often as a yoga teacher instructs a class to get out of their heads in an average class, particularly during standing forward folds.)

The relief and calm experienced by yoga students in and shortly after standing forward folds, especially when these poses are taken after more intense poses, is like the grin of the Cheshire Cat. At the end of the chapter, the Cheshire Cat vanishes slowly, leaving its grin to linger for some time. Similarly, the effects of a standing forward fold can linger long after the pose is over.

5-Minute Practice Overview
Standing Forward Folds

I let go of external desires and turn within myself.
My inner joy bursts out of my heart.
I find and access happiness from inside myself.

Gorilla

Fingers to Toes

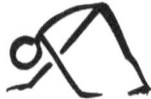

Pyramid

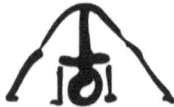

Straddle Fold

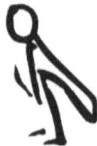

Squat

Fingers to Toes Pose

ASANA

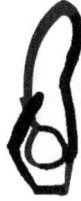

INTENTION

I can handle all details with ease.
I have a grip on details with an eye on the big picture.
I let the worries fall off my shoulders.
I am grounded with my fingers and toes to earth.
I let go of deep fears and anxieties that I hold in my hamstrings.
I am grounded and stable.

Gorilla Pose

ASANA

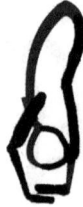

INTENTION

I am relaxed, calm, and peaceful.
I relax into what is and accept what happens.
I am able to let go of control and let things unfold naturally.

Pyramid Pose

ASANA

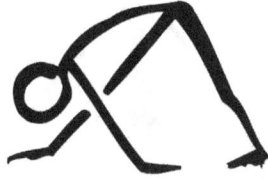

INTENTION

I am stable.
My life is mysterious, like a pyramid, mystical.
I honor my body as my temple.
I always have choices and options.
I access hidden aspects of myself and my life.

Straddle Forward Fold

ASANA

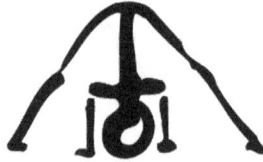

INTENTION

I am strong, steady, and well rooted.
From the support of gravity, I am light and buoyant.
I am relaxed and calm, surrendered and at ease.
I am soothed, calm, relaxed, surrendered and at peace.
I fold inside myself.
I drop my thoughts and rest in ease.
I drain my heart energy into my head.

Squat

ASANA

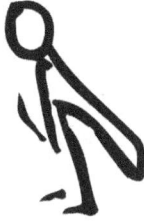

INTENTION

I am firmly planted and have a home here on planet Earth.
I let go, and find relief.
When I let go, I have room to expand and feel taller.
Spirit and Grace are always with me, through every form of release.

Off the Mat Trick
MOZI Method - Letting Go

Benefits

ASANA - released muscle tension in low back, shoulders & neck

INTENTION - clear mind & decreased over-thinking

SPIRIT - you will feel relaxed and released

ASANA - MOVE

- stand with your feet square & knees bent.
- Lay your belly on your thighs and drop your head.
- Shake your head and shoulders as they dangle below your heart
- Smile, a Cheshire Cat grin

INTENTION - THINK

- "I release and let go"
- "I let go of attachments"
- "I shake extra thoughts out of my head"

SPIRIT - BREATHE

Breathe out as you fold down. Breathe in as you shake and dangle.

Dosage

Practice this for 20-50 breaths a day, both when you need it and when you don't.

- 10 breaths when you wake up
- while waiting (I do it while waiting for gas to pump in my car)
- 5 breaths when you feel extra tight and tense
- 10 breaths before getting into bed

Standing Forward Folds
Journal

Date/Time:

Mood

      Body -

      Mind -

      Spirit -

Intention

Practice Summary

Insight

The Mad Hatter

Inverting Your Perspective
Inversions

There's Plenty of Room

There was a table set out under a tree in front of the house, and the March Hare and the Hatter were having tea at it: a Dormouse was sitting between them, fast asleep. . .The table was a large one, but the three were all crowded together at one corner of it:
"No room! No room!" they cried out when they saw Alice coming. "There's plenty of room!" said Alice indignantly, as she sat down in the large arm-chair at one end of the table.

In Chapter VII of *Alice's Adventures in Wonderland*, Alice meets the famous Mad Hatter and March Hare at a perpetual tea party with a sleeping mouse. She takes a seat at the table, despite being told there is no room. At this point, Alice has already accepted that things in Wonderland are upside-down and backwards. When she sits down, she asserts her right to be there. Alice now understands that the best way to engage in Wonderland is to play along with the madness.

"It wasn't very civil of you to sit down without being invited," said the March Hare. "it's laid for a great many more than three." said Alice.

In a yoga class, inversions are likely the most un-inviting portion of the practice because they appear dangerous, and the most physically challenging. The inversions require the yogi to essentially take their own seat, like Alice, at the madness table of the yoga practice. At the same time, if you play along, like Alice does, inversions are also somewhat enticing, sparking curiosity and play. Just like the Mad Hatter's tea table, yoga inversions come with all kinds of reasons not to try them (contraindications, fears, anxieties, and more). Yet, some yogis dive right in, with no fear, like Alice, ignoring the warnings and red flags and just "drinking the tea" so to speak.

For me, in my late twenties and early thirties, I played with inversions like a little kid dangling from my knees off the monkey bars of the playground. I didn't care if I fell, and I kept getting back up to try again and again and again. My ability to balance and stay steady, while it improved generally over time, seemed to shift arbitrarily from day to day. Some days I could land a handstand or headstand, and other days I would roll out time and time again. Later in my practice, after suffering several over-use injuries, I became more cautious and precise about inversions, using props and walls for support. While I have never really mastered the skill of balancing on my hands or standing on my head, getting my body upside-down, inverting my physical reality, has taught me many things about life.

> *"Then you should say what you mean," the March Hare went on.*
> *"I do," Alice hastily replied; "at least— I mean what I say— that's the same thing you know."*
> *"Not the same thing a bit!" said the Hatter. "Why, you might just as well say that 'I see what I eat' is the same thing as 'I eat what I see'!"*

At the Mad Hatter's tea table, the March Hare, the Dormouse, and the Mad Hatter play with the inverting language, pointing out that the inverse phrases have quite different meanings. They challenge Alice to be precise with her language and word choice, because inverted phrasing is most certainly not synonymous.

In yoga, standing upright is quite significantly different from being upside down. Turning your body upside down, be it in an Arm Balance, Headstand, or a variation of Shoulder Stand, is a means of both viewing things from a different perspective, and engaging physical muscles you don't often use. Inversions in yoga help you look at your situation in life from an inverted, slightly different, perspective, and activate different muscles and skills to navigate those experiences.

Yoga practice is an inversion of your life off the mat. Like the old adage, *as above, so below*, as in Heaven, so on Earth. The cliché "Heaven on Earth" is the inverted reality of yoga. When you are challenged to bring your head to the earth and your feet to the sky, you learn that the same principles of balance, alignment, structure, and architecture apply as when your feet are on the floor and your head is toward the sky. However, you must use your muscles differently than you are normally accustomed to using them. Inversions require an awareness of architecture from the root to the crown, from the base to the sky, from Heaven to Earth, and from Earth to Heaven.

> You might just as well say," added the March Hare, "that 'I like what I get" is the same thing as "I get what I like!"
> "You might just as well say," added the Dormouse, who seemed to be talking in his sleep, 'that 'I breathe when I sleep' is the same things as 'I sleep when I breathe'!"
> "It is the same thing with you," said the Hatter, and here the conversation dropped, and the party sat silent for a minute. . .

In Latin the word *invert* means *turn inward*. The inverted language at the tea-table eventually causes the Mad Hatter, Dormouse, and March Hare to fall silent, essentially forcing them to *turn within*. The force of gravity in yoga inversions make speech difficult, and cause a rush of blood to your head, making you think differently. Put simply, Inversions are one of the quickest ways to get you to shut up, turn inside yourself, and see things from a different perspective.

One such perspective shift Alice learns is how she looks at the concept of time. The tea-party attendees rotate around the very large table, like a clock, shifting seats whenever they feel like it, while at the same time, seemingly breaking all the rules of time. The Mad Hatter fidgets with a watch that tells the month but not the time, and the March Hare even dips the watch into his tea.

> "if you knew Time as well as I do," said the Hatter, "you wouldn't talk about wasting it. It's him."
> "I don't know what you mean," said Alice.
> "Of course you don't!" the Hatter said, tossing his head contemptuously. "I dare say you never even spoke to Time!"
> "Perhaps not," Alice cautiously replied: "but I know I have to beat time when I learn music."
> "Ah! that accounts for it," said the Hatter. "He won't stand beating. Now, if you only kept on good terms with him, he'd do almost anything you liked with the clock.

Here, Alice is challenged to think of Time as a *he* rather than an *it*. However, since ancient Greek times, and likely even before that, humans have personified Time into the character of Father Time, also known as Chronos, or Saturn. Father Time represents the flow of time and its effects. He is a reminder that time devours all things, and, like the sand in an hourglass, life eventually runs out. All things come to an end. But, this episode with the Mad Hatter implies the opposite is true in Wonderland. For the Mad Hatter, time is stuck at 6pm, tea-time, and he is condemned to rotate around a table, because once upon a time he "murdered time" while singing, and the Red Queen condemned him. In essence, the tea table turns Alice's perspective of time upside down, like turning over an hourglass.

Inversions in yoga practice have the same effect on my relationship with Time. While I'm in a balance pose or warrior pose, I often feel like time stands still, especially as I'm waiting for a teacher to call the next pose when I feel fatigue setting in. However, in inversions, I want to grab on to time. I want to hover in space and stay longer. When I do occasionally find the magical-just-right-place where I can balance on my hands or head, I want the sands of the hourglass to freeze.

However, like the personification of Father Time, all things come to an end. Everything eventually rots and decays in order to be re-born, like Father Time handing over his tools to Baby New Year each year.

It is interesting to note here that until now, Alice's experience of time in Wonderland has been in watching the White Rabbit fret about being late, constantly checking his pocket-watch. So even within Wonderland, the definition of Time is flexible.

My own upside-down perception of all this talk about Time is that Time is relevant mostly to our own relationship with the concept of Time. If we cultivate a healthy relationship with the concept of the passing of time, and we work in concert with Time to pass Time wisely, we have a more fulfilling experience of life. However, if we *waste* or *murder* or *beat* Time, we fall to the habits of being mindless in life and missing out. Time must be respected, in both his ability to pass and his ability to seemingly stay still.

Instead of circling the conversation and the table too much on the topic of Time, The March Hare suggests a story. The Dormouse complies by telling a story of three little sisters who live *well in* while living *in a well* of a treacle.

> *"and they drew all manner of things—everything that begins with an M—. . .such as mousetraps, and the moon, and memory, and muchness—you know you say things are 'much of a muchness'—did you ever see such a thing as a drawing of a muchness?"*

The final inversion of the chapter is the inversion of madness to muchness. In his story the Dormouse introduces the concept of muchness, and asks Alice for her perspective on muchness. When she tries to respond, the Mad Hatter scolds her, and she finally gets fed up with the rudeness of the Mad Hatter and leaves. Ultimately, Alice's homeland and Wonderland are inversions of each other. When she chooses to walk away from the *madness,* opting to leave *muchness* on the table, she notices a door leading into a tree. And her curiosity is opened once again. She finds herself back in the hall with the little door to the garden, where she eats bits of the mushroom that make her shrink, until she can fit the key in the door and enter the garden at last.

Like Alice, I finally got fed up with trying to find my *muchness* in the *madness* of perfecting inversions in yoga classes. Balancing on my hands and standing on my head, at some point, no longer seemed a valuable way to spend my time. It was when I stopped trying to be *muchness* and left the mad tea table of yoga teachers trying to tell me how to be and what to do that I found the beautiful garden of yoga that I now call Yoga Wonderland. While yes, I do occasionally play with inversions in my home practice now, I do so without an intention of mastery, but rather with that same child-like play I had as a kid dangling from my knees on the jungle gym.

5-Minute Practice Overview
Inversions

I find joy when things go upside down.
I am grounded even when the world goes wonky.
I can turn anything around as I need.

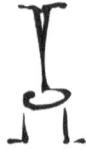

Handstand

Headstand

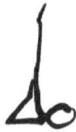

Shoulder Stand

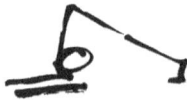

Plough

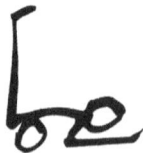

Legs up the Wall

Handstand

ASANA

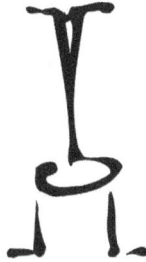

INTENTION

I am grounded in my actions and my decisions.
I stand tall in any circumstance.
I am strong and centered enough to hold myself stable anywhere.
I am centered.
I find joy in the moments when my world is upside down.

Headstand

ASANA

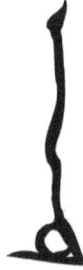

INTENTION

I am protected and safe to explore new perspectives in life.
I am in perfect alignment with my life purpose.
I am balanced, grounded, and free.
I am free from attachments, worries, and anxieties.
I embrace liberty, freedom and expression.

Shoulder Stand

ASANA

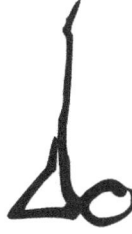

INTENTION

I stay safe.
I proceed with a full heart.
I express myself fully.
I drop burdens from my shoulders to Mother Earth.
I walk in vitality.
I balance my metabolism and sleep/wake cycles of life.

Plough

ASANA

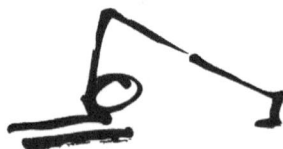

INTENTION

I look deep inside myself.
I am strong and stand tall, no matter what position I take.
No matter what situation I encounter, I am grounded.
I do my part and let the rest go.

Legs Up the Wall

ASANA

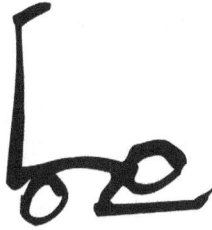

INTENTION

I am restored, renewed, and relaxed.
I no longer need to do the work.
Let it be.
I allow my worries and actions to drain into earth.
Mother Earth takes care of the details for me.

Off the Mat Trick
MOZI Method – Inversion

Benefits

> ASANA -ability to use all body muscles together
>
> INTENTION - increased determination and will
>
> SPIRIT - you will view your world from a different perspective

ASANA - MOVE

- Take rag-doll or forward fold while straddling a doorway, planting your hands on the ground on either side of the door-frame
- Push your back and neck into the door-frame so the frame lines with your spine between your shoulder blades
- Walk your feet up the door frame until one leg is straight up and the other leg stabilizes you

INTENTION - THINK

- "I turn my world upside down to see a different perspective"
- "I play with upside down perceptions."
- "I am safe and supported even when my world goes upside down"

SPIRIT - BREATHE

Breathe out as you push down into your hands. Breathe in as you lift your upper leg and push into the stabilizing foot.

Dosage

Practice this 1-3 x a day for 5-10 breaths

- 10 breaths when you wake up
- when walking through a doorway at home, pause for a handstand
- 10 breaths before getting into bed

Standing Forward Folds
Journal

Date/Time:

Mood

> Body -
> Mind -
> Spirit -

Intention

Practice Summary

Insight

The Queen's Croquet-Ground

Make Up Your Own Rules
Back Bends

A Very Curious Thing

A large rose-tree stood near the entrance of the garden: the roses growing on it were white, but there were three gardeners at it, busily painting them red. Alice thought this a very curious thing"

In Chapter VIII, Alice finally enters the beautiful garden, only to discover that it is not quite as beautiful as she expected. Yet, she maintains her mindset of curiosity, and her sense of self-confidence while engaged in conversation with these flimsy playing cards who have an even flimsier sense of logic.

"why, the fact is, you see, Miss, this here ought to have been a red rose-tree, and we put a white one in by mistake, and if the Queen was to find it out, we should all have our heads cut off, you know."

Alice has entered the land of the Queen of Hearts, who seemingly doesn't have a heart of her own as she threatens at every turn to have someone or other be-headed. Her orders are never actually carried out, at least not as Alice is able to see, but the threats are enough to send everyone scurrying about and tip-toeing around the moods and whims of the Queen.

""The Queen! The Queen!"
and the three gardeners instantly threw themselves flat upon their faces. . . Alice was rather doubtful whether she ought not to lie down on her face like the three gardeners.

The first step in the backbend (heart-opening) series of the yoga poses is to lie, belly down to the earth in preparation for poses like cobra, locust, sphinx and bow. This position is actually the *pranam* or a full bow in reverence. It is done in many spiritual traditions, in offering to a guru or saint. In Alice's case, it is done by the gardeners out of fear of the Queen of Hearts.

"What's your name, child?"

"My name is Alice, so please your Majesty," said Alice very politely; but she added, to herself, "Why, they're only a pack of cards, after all. I needn't be afraid of them!"

Energetically, the full expression of a backbend is also the full expression of compassion and loving kindness, something completely foreign to the Queen of Hearts in Wonderland. As you go through your life, you may be faced with any number of people like the Queen. In yoga, (backbends especially) to open our hearts is quite a daunting task, especially when we face individuals with demeanors similar to the Queen of Hearts in Wonderland. At the same time, it is necessary to protect ourselves from attack, and still keep our hearts open for compassion, no matter what. The spiritual practice of yoga helps us look through outside appearances to the purity of Spirit inside all of us, and to behave accordingly.

In this scene, Alice chooses to respond to the Queen respectfully, while also affirming to herself that she is not afraid of them as they are only a pack of cards. She does not believe the Queen can hurt her.

In yoga, practitioners are often prone to over-do backbends. They fail to engage their core strength enough to protect the spine, and thus end up folding on their spines and causing compression injuries, particularly in the low back. When Alice chooses to be respectful to the Queen, she opens her heart like a backbend to the Queen. But, when she affirms silently to herself that the furious Queen cannot hurt her, her intention is symbolic of engaging her core to protect her spine in backbends.

It is essential, when being kind and compassionate, and caring to for others, to consider yourself and your own needs first, to protect yourself, to keep yourself safe while still be open.

The Queen turned crimson with fury, and, after glaring at her for a moment like a wild beast, began screaming, "Off with her head! Off—"

"Nonsense!" said Alice, very loudly and decidedly, and the Queen was silent.

In this scene, Alice finds new courage that she hasn't expressed before. She becomes the only being in Wonderland to demand respect from the Queen and to stand up to her rants, rendering the Queen speechless. Eventually, other creatures, including the Queen, begin to look up to Alice for answers. In doing so, Alice engaged her core and stood up for her own protections and strength first. As soon as she does, the Queen is silenced, and diverts her attention elsewhere. Just as in backbends. If you feel the slightest twinge, ache or pinch, engaging your core, asserting your right to protect yourself, choosing not to give too much away, you will eliminate any danger. This works both physically in your body and relationally with others.

Interesting then, that the most common injury in yoga that results from the heart-opening energy of back-bends is not heart-break, but rather, BACK-break. In essence, we break our backs from bending over backward for people, giving too much, and not taking care of ourselves.

Practicing backbends and heart opening in your body and in life requires extreme mindfulness in walking that careful line between serving others and taking care of your own needs. You must first take care of yourself before serving others because if you serve others first, you will deplete yourself, creating resentment and failed connection in relationship.

"I see!" said the Queen, who had meanwhile been examining the roses. "Off with their heads!" and the procession moved on, three of the soldiers remaining behind to execute the unfortunate gardeners, who ran to Alice for protection.

"You shan't be beheaded!" said Alice, and she put them into a large flower-pot that stood near. The three soldiers wandered about for a minute or two, looking for them, and then quietly marched off after the others.

"Are their heads off?" shouted the Queen.

"Their heads are gone, if it please your Majesty!" the soldiers shouted in reply.

Alice steps in to rescue the three gardeners. She opens her heart to serve the gardeners, knowing in her own confidence that it won't hurt her at all. In turn, the soldiers play along as well. Heart energy is contagious! Alice opens her heart, and the soldiers do as well. In fact, when the Queen asks to confirm the beheading, the soldiers don't even *really* lie. They simply tell her their heads are gone, which is true. The soldiers couldn't find the heads to cut them off, so they were in fact, *gone*.

Here's where things get really curious! In yoga, the Sanskrit word for the heart chakra is *anahata* which translates to mean "that which can never be broken." The Queen of Hearts in Wonderland inadvertently emphasizes this concept because no one in Wonderland is ever really beheaded! While there are threats, and everyone runs around fearful of the potential, the actual beheadings never really happen. Perhaps this is symbolic of the fact that the human emotional heart never really breaks.

While we often speak of being broken-hearted, the truth is that when we are emotionally hurt, the human heart never really *breaks*. Physically, the heart is made of tissue that is pliable, malleable, bendable, so it doesn't *break*. Rather, it just stretches and tears, and eventually heals itself back up again. Like any other tissue in the body, when stretched and torn, albeit painful, it stitches itself back up stronger than before. Thus, heart-ache only creates a stronger heart to be more open to love and compassion and kindness in the future.

> *"Come on then!" roared the Queen, and Alice joined the procession, wondering very much what would happen next.*

Alice maintains her sense of curiosity as she follows the procession to a croquet-ground. However, with all the equipment being played by living beings, the whole game is utter chaos.

> *the croquet-balls were live hedgehogs, and the mallets live flamingoes, and the soldiers had to double themselves up and stand on their hands and feet, to make the arches. . . Alice soon came to the conclusion that it was a very difficult game indeed. . .*

"I don't think they play at all fairly," Alice began, in rather a complaining tone, "and they all quarrel so dreadfully one can't hear one's-self speak—and they don't seem to have any rules in particular; at least, if there are, nobody attends to them—and you've no idea how confusing it is all the things being alive"...

The Queen's Croquet-Ground is symbolic of the human game of Love. All the players involved are living beings, and some are used as tools against others. Everyone scurries about playing by their own rules. The worst of the game occurs when the Queen (an irrational woman) comes in threatening to chop the heads off all the players. The game itself is symbolic of the old adage *all's fair in love and war.*

Discouraged by the chaos of the game, Alice is distracted by the Cheshire Cat as a head with no body. When the Queen orders the Cheshire Cat to be executed, an argument ensues about how to cut the head off a creature that has no body. In essence, the Cheshire Cat , symbolic of an un-attached ego, beats the Queen at her own game by making up rules that don't match the Queen's.

Perhaps the lesson that the Cheshire Cat is suggesting is that the way to "win" the game of life and love is to detach your ego from the process entirely and refuse to play by the rules of others, but rather, to play by the rules of your own making.

When people around you appear to be playing a game without following any rules, like the Queen's croquet match, it is your responsibility to find the place inside yourself where forgiveness, sweetness, and connectedness win out over resentment, anger, and depression. This place already exists inside your heart. While the Queen's Heart is as two- dimensional as a playing card, allowing for only action or execution, Alice's heart, like all human hearts, is multi-dimensional.

At the center of your heart, beneath all the energetic layers of physicality, relationship, self-love, and otherness, is a place where you are one with Spirit. Like the vanishing Cheshire Cat, the *anahata* is unable to be executed, injured, or harmed in any way. The backbends of yoga, often considered the climax of the practice, serve to feed your heart physically and energetically, while reminding you of your own *anahata* center.

5-Minute Practice Overview
Back Bends

I love unconditionally.
I open myself to the greater wisdoms that live deep within me.

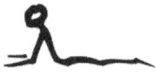 Sphinx

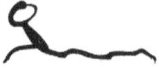 Cobra

Locust

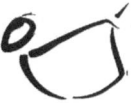 Bow

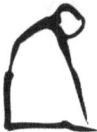 Camel

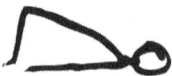 Bridge

Sphinx

ASANA

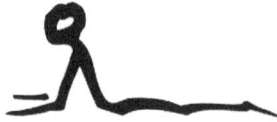

INTENTION

I am safe and supported in my vulnerability.
I have the wisdom of an oracle within me.
I am open to receiving healing and wisdom.
I am perfect just as I am today.
I open gradually, at just the right pace for myself.
My service to others comes first from my heart and then from action.

Cobra

ASANA

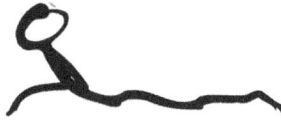

INTENTION

I love myself unconditionally.
I lead with my heart.
I am strong as I face change.
I am humble.
I shed my skin and transform with grace.

Locust Pose

ASANA

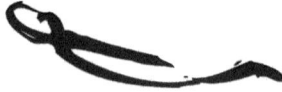

INTENTION

I am strong and solid as I open my heart.
I express love for myself and others.
I have natural fluidity as I move through life.
I am forgiving and understanding.

Bow Pose

ASANA

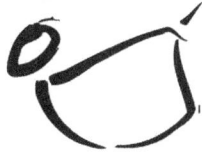

INTENTION

I have gained wisdom from my past to bring to my present.
I am guided by past experiences.
I am on the right course.
I let go, with careful action and right aim.
I am held by the grace of Spirit.

Camel Pose

ASANA

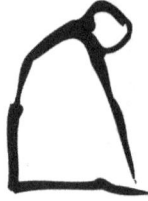

INTENTION

I am flexible because I am strong.
I am humble.
I am calm, centered, balanced, stable, and safe through my journey.
I am strong enough to make it through any challenge.
I can accomplish the seemingly impossible.
I am prepared for any drought in my life.
I am able to let go of control and trust in the guidance of Spirit.
I am open to receive the blessings of Spirit.

Bridge Pose

ASANA

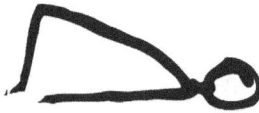

INTENTION

I am open to transition and change in my life.
I walk the bridge from here to there with ease.
I am comfortable in the space between.
I let my challenges be water under the bridge.
Through love, I heal conflict in any relationship.
I can be the bridge in relationship and connection.

Off the Mat Trick
MOZI Method – Heart Opening

Benefits

> ASANA - improved function of lungs & heart, relaxed shoulders
> INTENTION -increased sense of openness and expansion
> SPIRIT - you will have better relationships

ASANA - MOVE

- Hold your hands like you're holding a lunch tray, elbows in at your ribs.
- Face your palms up
- Point your forearms out from your torso at 45 degree angles
- Plug your elbows into your ribs to slightly engage your core
- Feel your breastbone open as your shoulder blades flatten on your back

INTENTION - THINK

- "I open to possibilities."
- "I am compassionate and loving towards others"
- "I protect myself as I open to relationship with others"

SPIRIT - BREATHE

Breathe in as you open your chest. Breathe out as you relax your shoulders.

Dosage

Practice this 1-3 x a day for 5-10 breaths
- 10 breaths when you wake up
- 5 breaths before engaging with a difficult person in your life
- 10 breaths before getting into bed

Standing Back Bends
Journal

Date/Time:

Mood

        Body -

        Mind -

        Spirit -

Intention

Practice Summary

Insight

The Moral Duchess

Everything's Got a Moral
Hip Openers

Everything's Got a Moral

"You can't think how glad I am to see you again, you dear old thing!" said the Duchess, as she tucked her arm affectionately into Alice's, and they walked off together. . . "You're thinking about something, my dear, and that makes you forget to talk. I can't tell you just now what the moral of that is, but I shall remember it in a bit."

"Everything's got a moral, if only you can find it."

In Chapter IX of *Alice's Adventures in Wonderland*, Alice meets up with The Duchess, who pulls Alice away from the Queen's croquet game. The Duchess accuses Alice of forgetting to speak while at the same time instructing Alice that everything that happens has a moral or lesson to absorb. Ironically, as the Duchess is reprimanding Alice for her silence, Alice is contemplating one of the morals of life. Right after Alice links arms with the Duchess, Alice goes silent as she gets lost in thought (day-dreaming) about how foods such as pepper and vinegar and sweet things impact a person's temperament.

Just like in regular school, each time a child is caught 'day-dreaming' (which is really a form of meditation), s/he is called back to attention to class, much like the Duchess discouraging Alice for thinking for herself. Perhaps day-dreaming should be encouraged in certain circumstances because it is a process of turning deep within yourself to access those still small voice wisdoms that are ultimately the "morals in everything" type Truths with a capital T.

In yoga, the hip openers part of practice are where you are completely ready to receive the "morals in everything" wisdoms that occur through day-dreaming. During hip openers, the energy of the room usually goes quite still and quiet. During this time, students are fully able to turn in on themselves and hear the wisdoms that live within themselves. As all the other clutter and energies have been cleaned out through earlier poses in the practice, the hip openers tend to be the part of practice where intuitive insights make themselves known and clear.

In my own practice, I have found that the hip openers series is where I get the best ideas and insights. In fact, I have come to keep a small journal next to my mat so that I can sit up from half or double pigeon to jot down a few words to remind myself of the insights I received. Some of my most brilliant article and book ideas have come out during hip openers, not to mention some of the greatest insights about my own life and process. Everything has got a moral. Everything happened for a reason, if only you can find it. Hip openers is the time in the practice when we are able to dig through the deeper layers of life and find the wisdom and insights that lead to the morals and reasons for things that occur in the world.

Perhaps it is the silent quality of hip openers combined with the forward fold action that allows me to turn inside myself, quiet and still the excess flutterings of my thoughts and see the deeper still small voice in myself. When I'm in yoga classes, I often find myself wishing the teacher would stop talking and just let me think. Silence is Golden. I catch myself yoga-day-dreaming and disengaging from the language of the teacher entirely. For this reason, I have made it a practice in my own teaching to encourage my students to listen to their own thoughts while I go silent as a teacher to allow time for my students to yoga-day-dream.

> *"The game's going on rather better now," she said, by way of keeping up the conversation a little.*
> *Tis' so," said the Duchess: "Oh, 'tis love, 'tis love, that makes the world go round!"*
> *"Somebody said," Alice whispered, "that it's done by everybody minding their own business!"*
> *"Ah, well! It means much the same thing," said the Duchess, digging her sharp little chin into Alice's shoulder as she added, "and the moral of that is—'Take care of the sense, and the sounds will take care of themselves.'"*

When Alice does come out of her day-dream and engages in conversation with the Duchess, she becomes an observer to the outside world of the game of croquet. She notices that the game goes better when everyone does their own things for themselves ("it's done by everybody minding their own business!")

Alice sees things differently now, having had a chance to *really* listen to herself. She is no longer caught up in the drama of everything else and that outside herself. As such, she is able to access her intuition, her insight, and her own perspective better.

While many of the morals of the Duchess are rambling nonsense, occasionally a gem of wisdom escapes her lips. For example: "Take care of the sense, and the sounds will take care of themselves." The moral here is that when you step outside the external drama of what is happening *to* you and turn in on yourself and pay attention to how you FEEL (your sense) on your inside, then the sounds (how you heal) will take care of itself.

A common phrase yoga teachers use during intense parts of practice is *"you must feel in order to heal."* Hip openers are such a deeply physical experience that they force the yogi to be fully present to themselves (feel), paying attention to both what they feel physically, and the insights they are processing mentally and emotionally as a result (heal).

> You must feel
> (take care of the sense)
> in order to heal
> (and the sounds will take care of themselves).

When your body goes through a physical trauma like a major accident or fall, it goes into a state of shock as a protective mechanism. Shock turns down the volume of the pain at the time of the injury, because otherwise it is too intense to handle. Then, over time, through the healing process, the pain sneaks out in manageable doses. Full healing is not complete until the pain of the full experience has been felt.

The same kind of healing process occurs when you experience an emotional trauma, and usually a physical trauma and an emotional trauma occur at the same time.

Energetically, when you go through emotional trauma (loss, grief, moving, losing a job, etc.) your energy goes into a similar state of shock, hiding the intense emotions so as to not overwhelm your body. As the emotional issues of our lives live inside the physical tissues of our bodies, the pain of emotional trauma usually resides and hides inside the tissues of the hips and pelvis. Your hips and pelvis are shaped like a bowl, intended to *hold,* and they also house the densest and strongest muscles, ligament, and tendon tissues of your body that are most capable of holding the heaviest loads. The more emotional baggage you hold onto in your life, the tighter your hips may be.

While prescription medications and narcotics can effectively mask physical pain, and anti-depressants and mood stabilizers may mask emotional pain, neither form of pharmaceutical medication will effectively release the physical and/or emotional pain to promote full healing. They are necessary to prevent the deepest pain when you are not in a place to safely feel it. But eventually, you must FEEL in order to fully HEAL. When used improperly, drugs become an addictive support system for the human tendency is to shove pain back into its hiding place rather than let it release.

The hip openers serve as a way to open the door to let the baggage of past trauma release, come out, and encourage you to FEEL the pains and process them through so that you may HEAL. The human tendency during Hip Openers is to try to identify reasons and explanations for the emotions and sensations that arise, just like the Duchess finding the morals in everything.

5-Minute Practice Overview
Hip Openers

I am open to spiritual wisdom and insight.
My inner thoughts and feels matter.

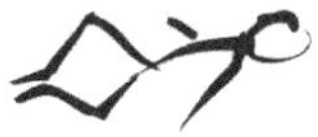
Reclined Butterfly

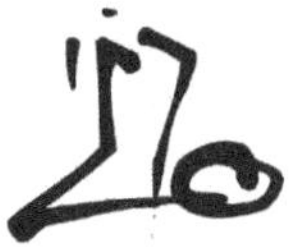
Dead Bug

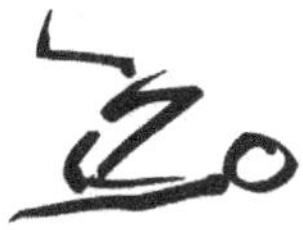
Reclined Pigeon

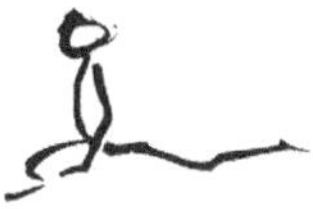
Half Pigeon

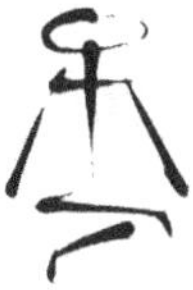
Double Pigeon

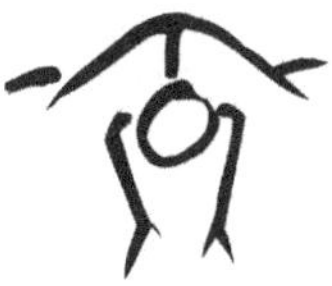
Frog

Reclined Butterfly

ASANA

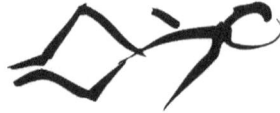

INTENTION

Like the caterpillar before it becomes a butterfly, I begin close to the
ground, connected to earth.
I am bound together at the center of my soul.
I am exquisitely beautiful.
I love myself through the massive changes and transitions of life.

Happy Baby Pose
(Dead Bug)

ASANA

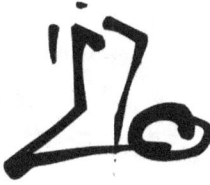

INTENTION

I am naturally supported, as if lying on a bed of leaves.
Even in pain, good pain, I access the joy of a baby.
I am relaxed and calm.
I let GO!

Reclined Pigeon

ASANA

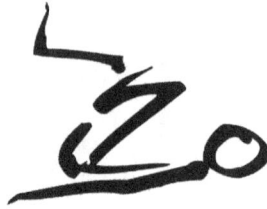

INTENTION

I am adaptable to new circumstances.
I have the endurance to journey through long challenges.
I am a survivor who gets through even the most extreme conditions.
I am a messenger of hope.
I am a harbinger of love and light in a new life.

Half Pigeon

ASANA

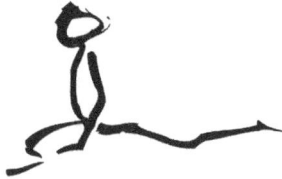

INTENTION

I am at home in my body.
I am safe, despite the chaos I may feel.
I release old patterns and past traumas.
I love myself exactly as I am.
I am open to intuitive wisdom.

Double Pigeon

ASANA

INTENTION

I am safe.
I am prepared for the unknown.
There is always a place of flexibility in my body and life.
I look deep inside myself to face my wounds and release my gifts.

Frog Pose

ASANA

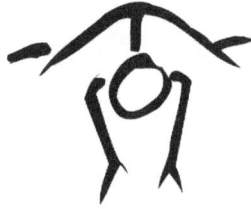

INTENTION

I feel safe and loved on my soft bed of props.
Like a frog, I have a kick and buoyancy in my spirit.
I support myself.
I let go.
I am safe.

Off the Mat Trick
MOZI Method - Feeling to Heal

Benefits

ASANA - softens hand, wrist, and elbow pain

INTENTION -more open mindedness and go with the flow thoughts

SPIRIT - you will let go of things that have held you back

ASANA - MOVE

- Hold your hands in a fist (keeping a grip)
- Open your hands slowly as you imagine those things being released (letting them heal)

INTENTION - THINK

- "I feel in order to heal."
- "I let go of that which I no longer need"
- "I let go of past issues, traumas, and experiences to open myself to what's new and next"

SPIRIT - BREATHE

Breathe in as you close your hand in a fist.

Breathe out as you open your hand to receive.

Dosage

Practice this 1-3 x a day for 5-10 breaths

- 10 breaths when you wake up
- 5 breaths when you are triggered by past trauma and anxieties
- 10 breaths before getting into bed

Hip Openers
Journal

Date/Time:

Mood

      Body -

      Mind -

      Spirit -

Intention

Practice Summary

Insight

The Mock Turtle
& The Gryphon

Lessen the Lessons
Seated Forward Folds

Tell Your History

"Have you seen the Mock Turtle yet?"
"No," said Alice. "I don't even know what a Mock Turtle is."
"It's the thing Mock Turtle Soup is made from,"
said the Queen.
"I never saw one, or heard of one," said Alice.
"Come on then," said the Queen,
"and he shall tell you his history."
They very soon came upon a Gryphon lying fast asleep in the sun. . . "Up, lazy thing!" said the Queen,
"and take this young lady to see the Mock Turtle, and to hear his history."

In chapters IX and X, as Alice engages with the Gryphon and the Mock Turtle, she gets a lesson in paradox. She is faced with two characters who are on opposite ends of the spectrum in terms of their capacity to express emotions.

"What fun!" said the Gryphon, half to itself, half to Alice.
"What is the fun?" said Alice.
"Why, she, "said the Gryphon. "It's all her fancy, that: they never executes nobody, you know. Come on!". . .
So they went up to the Mock Turtle, who looked at them with large eyes full of tears, but said nothing. . .
said the Mock Turtle in a deep, hollow tone:
"sit dow both of you, and don't speak a word till I've finished."

Alice has just come from just come from the contradiction of the Queen's croquet match where virtually everyone was condemned to death, but the King pardons everyone. The Gryphon, who is remarkably amused by the circumstances around him, introduces Alice to the Mock Turtle, who speaks in sighs and sobs, even as he perpetually denies that he is sad. She is challenged to learn how to live in the presence of these paradoxical opposites.

Yoga, in its core definition, is the practice of recognizing the inherent union of two opposites, like the yin/yang. The word yoga comes from the root word *yuj* which translates to mean *yoke*. As we live in a dualistic world of day and night, dark and light, we are conditioned to believe in opposing forces, black and white. Yoga practice helps you to value both sides of the coin, and acknowledge that two opposites make a whole and are part of the full existence. In essence, then, you can have a fuller experience of life when you can, say, experience opposite like happiness and sadness at the same time.

By this point of the story, Alice has been offered so many oddities that she is able to grasp the concept of non-duality, that opposites do not necessarily need to be mutually exclusive. Rather, they can coexist quite naturally. The Mock Turtle represents sadness, and the Gryphon represent joy. In conversation with them both, Alice learns the value of experiencing both. Non-duality.

In yoga forward folds, it is easier to perform a stretch that many yoga teachers call *dual-action*. For example, when you push your heels of your legs, while simultaneously pulling on your heels with your hands, you access a dual-action stretch inside your legs and spine that cannot be touched with only one force. The equal and opposite force of pushing and pulling at the same time touches something deep inside. In my own practice, I do find that I can practice dual-action push-pull stretches in any pose of a sequence, but in these longer quiet holding stretches, I can more easily access the equal and opposite forces in my body than in standing poses where I'm concerned about balance and strength.

So, they sat down, and nobody spoke for some minutes. .
.
"once," said the Mock Turtle at least, with a deep sigh, "I was a real Turtle."
These words were followed by a very long silence, broken only by an occasional exclamation of "Hjekrrh!" from the Gryphon, and the constant heavy sobbing of the Mock Turtle. Alice was very nearly getting up and saying, "Thank you, sir, for your interesting story," but she could not help thinking there must by more to come, so she sat still and said nothing.

The Mock Turtle offers even longer silences in his story than the Caterpillar did. Alice has learned patience and is curious enough to stick around to hear what the Mock Turtle might share. At this point, she has learned the golden value of silence, and has become comfortable in sitting in silence.

The deep silence of the seated forward folds is almost a squeeze of the deeper wisdoms that lives inside us, pushing them out into expression and communication. As the Mock Turtle is silent, he does eventually speak, and his story has power. Again, a paradox exists. Silence creates expression, and a more authentic communication. For me as a writer, as I turn deeply silent and still and fold in on myself in yoga forward folds, I gain insights and inspirations that make me want to write and speak and be heard. The deep silence and introspection of the fold actually inspires and motivates me to speak out and express. I often come out of forward folds feeling almost itchy and anxious to write or teach.

"We called him Tortoise because he taught us,". . . *"I only took the regular course."*

"Reeling and Writhing, of course, to begin with," the Mock Turtle replied: "and then the different branches of Arithmetic— Ambition, Distraction, Uglification, and Derision."

"Well, there was Mystery. . . ancient and modern, with Seaography: then Drawling—the Drawling-master was an old conger-eel, that used to come once a week: he taught us Drawling, Stretching, and Fainting in Coils."

The Mock Turtle and the Gryphon describe their school courses using plays on words such as 'reeling' and 'writhing' and 'drawling'. They also suggest that their schooling included courses about living life, not just acquiring skills. Alice is very curious about their schooling as it is so different from her own, as they studied things that she experienced in Wonderland, such as ambition, distraction, laughing and grief.

Most people stumble into yoga much like Alice stumbled into Wonderland, without really knowing what they are getting into. While Alice followed a White Rabbit out of curiosity, most yogis take their first class in search of some better quality of life. Like Alice, once in Wonderland, all the mysteries of yoga become very curious and intriguing. By the time you reach the floor series of poses towards the end of class, you are realizing that yoga is not just about stretching, but it is a school in Truth. The lessons you learn are far different than anything you learned in traditional academia, and far more valuable.

When I stepped on my yoga mat the first time, I wanted a way to stretch out after an intense cardio-kickboxing class. What I didn't realize was that my yoga mat was a rabbit hole of deeper life lessons and spiritual discoveries.

I remember vividly in my early days of practice, sighing deeply in seated forward fold, my face pressed into my knees, the backs of my thighs stretching in ways I'd never felt before. What was different about that stretch than any other time I had "touched my toes" was that I felt things inside myself, both physically and emotionally, that I always knew were there but had never felt before. The stretch in my legs wasn't just the muscles next to the skin, I felt something tug at bone depth. In as much, I also felt something deeply emotional in that stretch. The stretch of *something* close to my thigh bone felt like a chord of string deep inside my soul was being plucked, and tuned, and awakened. There was both a deep tension and a zinging tingle, a paradox of feels. It was that first deep stretch that I realized yoga was so much more than just a way to stay limber. It was a way to really access the depth of my being and connect my physical body to my soul essence.

For a time thereafter, I felt like my entire education had wronged me, by leaving huge gaps in my learning. I felt like everything I had ever learned in any class was, well, superficial. I wanted depth, but it was like my formal education had left me with an ability to articulate anything with any substance. Now, I do value my education, as it taught me my alphabet and vocabulary, and much more. Formal schooling leaves out so many important parts of Truth that Alice found in Wonderland, and I found in Yoga Wonderland, mainly in forward fold poses.

"And how many hours a day did you do lessons?" said Alice, in a hurry to change the subject.
"Ten hours the first day," said the Mock Turtle: "nine the

next, and so on."
What a curious plan!" exclaimed Alice.
"That's the reason they're called lessons," the Gryphon
remarked: "because they lessen from day to day."

As everything is upside-down and backwards in Wonderland, Alice is not surprised to find out that education is inside-out as well. In Wonderland, the goal is to study less, and experience more. The lessons LESSEN. While the Mock Turtle and Gryphon only speak of the lessons lessening in length of time, I might argue that they also lessen in instruction as well.

I was in a seated twist pose during a self-guided home practice once when I realized that a huge part of my yoga learning is about UN-Learning. I had to put away a lot of the things I had learned as ultimate truths in my formal education because they were limiting to the greater reality I was experiencing on my mat. Yoga taught me to un-learn, and to realize the value of not knowing what I don't know. I even had to un-learn a lot of the things my yoga teachers had taught me about practice because when I practice by myself, there was so much more that my yoga teachers had never shared. As I tried to teach these things to my own students, I realized many of them were wisdoms that cannot be taught. They must be felt. Experienced. Accessed on your own. Self-discovered. There is magic to self-discovery that does not exist under the guidance of a teacher.

When I first starting practicing yoga, like I did with formal education, the more I did, the more I wanted to do. I started with an hour practice once a week, which quickly became several times a week, which then evolved into trainings and retreats and workshops. There was a time when I sometimes did 18 hours of yoga in a day (I don't recommend this). But, in recent years, my practice, like the Mock Turtle's and Gryphon's has been lessening. What was once 1-3 hours a day is now 20-30 minutes a day, sometimes less. Yet, I find that the LESS I do, with more intention and mindfulness, the less I need. I feel healthier and stronger and more spiritually connected now than I did when I was attending 4-5 intensive trainings a year and practicing 3-5 hours a day. IN just ten minutes of my Yoga Wonderland practice now, I gain MORE insight and wisdom from myself than I ever did workshops, classes, and retreats.

> *"I could tell you my adventures—beginning from this morning," said Alice a little timidly: "but it's no use going back to yesterday, because I was a different person then."*
> *"Explain all that," said the Mock Turtle.*
> *"No, no! the adventures first," said the Gryphon in an impatient tone: "explanations take such a dreadful time."*

The Mock Turtle and the Gryphon ask Alice to share her own adventures with them. She stumbles to tell her story and admits that her experiences in Wonderland have changed her so much that she is not the same person she was yesterday.

Anyone who commits to a yoga practice will admit that it changes us. And, when you commit to a home practice and turn in on yourself in forward folds, you discover all the layers of yourself can co-exist.

5-Minute Practice Overview
Seated Forward Folds

The answers lie within me.
I don't know what I don't know.
I am open to connecting all things as ONE.

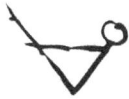 Boat Pose

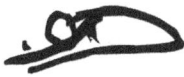 Seated Forward Fold

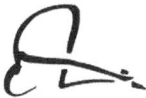 Tortoise

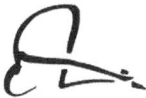 Rabbit Pose

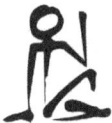 Seated Twist

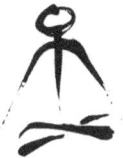 Lotus

Boat Pose

ASANA

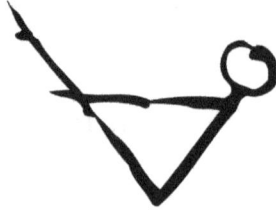

INTENTION

I float through any situation with grace.
I lift myself toward Heaven.
I am strong.
I am open to whatever course I may need to navigate.
I am relaxed, as if floating on the sea.

Seated Forward Fold

ASANA

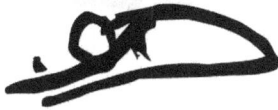

INTENTION

I am safe.
I nurture myself in many ways.
I take things EASY.
I am awake and aware, even when turning within.
I love myself.
I hand over my worries to Spirit.

Tortoise Pose

ASANA

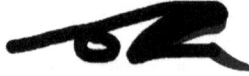

INTENTION

I am supported and open at the same time.
I can turn my eyes away from the race and focus on the journey.
Slow and steady wins my race.
I am strong enough to carry the heavy loads of my life.
Mother Earth holds my heart.

Rabbit Pose

ASANA

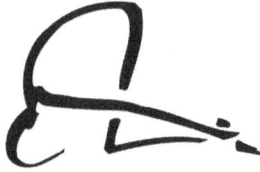

INTENTION

I trust my intuition to take me where I need to go.
Sometimes it is safe to stay still.
Sometimes it is best to flee.
Some fear is good fear.
A magical, mystical Wonderland lives inside me.

Seated Twist

ASANA

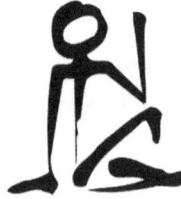

INTENTION

I am stable and supported.
I twist myself open to new possibilities, like opening a bottle.
I expand my awareness.
I maintain perspective in all situations.

Lotus Pose

ASANA

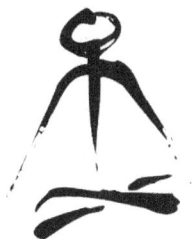

INTENTION

I am grounded.
I accept things just as they are.
My soul, and soles of my feet, are exposed and open.
Being myself is natural and easy.

Off the Mat Trick
MOZI Method – Speak Your Mind

Benefits

ASANA - releases neck and shoulder tension

INTENTION - connects your brain thoughts to your heart feelings

SPIRIT - you will speak your mind more clearly

ASANA - MOVE

- Tuck your chin slightly so your head is level
- Pull the back of your head back
- Align your earlobes over your shoulders
- Gaze at the horizon
- Bobble your head slightly to soften your neck muscles

INTENTION - THINK

- "I speak my mind."
- "I align my head and my heart"
- "I think and feel clearly"

SPIRIT - BREATHE

Focused Breathing

Dosage

Practice this 1-3 x a day for 5-10 breaths

- 10 breaths when you wake up
- 5 breaths when you have to speak your mind clearly to someone
- 10 breaths before getting into bed

Seated Forward Folds
Journal

Date/Time:

Mood

     Body -

     Mind -

     Spirit -

Intention

Practice Summary

Insight

The King, Queen & Knave

The Importance of Un-Importance
Final Rest

Evidence & Trial

The White Rabbit blew three blasts on the trumpet, and then unrolled the parchment scroll, and read as follows
"The Queen of Hearts, she mad some tarts,
All on a summer day:
The Knave of Hearts, he stole those tarts,
And took them quite away!"

In Chapters XI and XII of *Alice's Adventures in Wonderland,* Alice is brought to court, where the Knave is being tried for stealing the Queen's tarts. While the King serves as a tyrannical judge, the jurors write down random things; some even forget their own names. All the characters Alice has met in Wonderland, The White Rabbit, Little Bill, the March Hare, the Dormouse, the Mad Hatter, play various roles at the trial.

The purpose of the final rest (savasana) in yoga is to take some time to allow your body and nervous system to process all the things you have done in your practice. Like a jury trial, it is a time for your body to recount the events, your body parts to bear witness to what they experienced, and make judgements and determinations as to how to behave and function from here on out. Ideally, savasana is equal to ten percent of the total time of the practice, a time for the nervous system to run and process, and most importantly, settle.

Just at this moment, Alice felt a very curious sensation, which puzzled her a good deal until she made out what it was: she was beginning to grow larger again, and she thought at first she would get up and leave the court: but on second thoughts she decided to remain where she was as long as there was room for her.

When she first arrives at court, Alice is happy with the familiarity of it. She recognizes the elements of the court as the same as what she had learned about courts in school. After all the changes she experienced in

Wonderland, she is now pleased to be able to integrate what she knew from her life to what she had experienced in Wonderland.

As yogis settle into corpse pose, savasana, the familiarity of laying still and flat on the mat without having to perform any complex contortions is a great relief. At the same time, the nervous system is busy processing all the new information gathered during the practice. Just as Alice knows she cannot go back to yesterday and cannot be who she was before she entered Wonderland, yogis know that at the end of practice, the body is different, and cannot be like it was before.

The effects of eating the mushroom and drinking the potions begin to wear off and Alice starts to grow back to her natural size, she has the urge to get up and leave. Yet, on second thought, she decides to stay as long as she can. This urge to leave is very common for yogis in savasana as well. They often get antsy to be done with practice and get back to their every day lives. However, they also have so enjoyed their time on the mat that they don't want to leave. Like Alice, they find a place of being content in the eagerness to leave with the desire and curiosity to stay.

> *Imagine her surprise, when the White Rabbit read out, at the top of his shrill little voice, the name "Alice!"*
>
> *"Here!" cried Alice, quite forgetting in the flurry of the moment how large she had grown in the last few minutes, and she jumped up in such a hurry that she tipped over the jury-box with the edge of her skirt, upsetting all the jury-men on to the heads of the crowd below. . .*
>
> *"The trial cannot proceed," said the King in a very grave voice, "until all the jurymen are back in their proper places."*

When Alice gets up to go to the witness chair, she knocks over the jury box. While up until this point in the story, every episode has been about how Wonderland and the various characters of Wonderland have had an impact on Alice, this small scene shows that as a whole, Alice has an even more dramatic impact on Wonderland. Alice is a co-creator in a new reality for herself. Wonderland had an impact on her, but she had to be a willing participant, and in so doing, she had an impact on the world of Wonderland.

As I said earlier, savasana, the final resting pose of yoga is about integrating all the experiences you have had on your mat into a new state of existence for yourself. Yoga Wonderland has had an impact on you, and as a result, when you rise from savasana and re-engage with your world, you realize the greater impact you have on your world, just be virtue of your authentic being. Just as Alice is changed by Wonderland and Wonderland is changed by Alice, you are changed by yoga, and your world is changed by you.

At the end of most yoga classes, the teacher often closes the class with the blessing *namasté,* which loosely translates to "the light in me honors the light in you." While the practice of yoga is ultimately about recognizing the oneness in everything, the real test (or trial) of the practice is if you can apply what you learn on your mat to your every day life. As yoga influences you to have a deeper understanding of life, can you then go out into the world and influence the world around you? Can you impact the people around you as much or more than the yoga has impacted you? Namasté is a blessing and a greeting that honors and recognizes that we are all made up of neurological wiring that is impacted and influenced by everything and everyone we experience and encounter, while at the same time, we have that same impact and influence on others. To practice namasté is to emerge from the "trial" of yoga with a better understanding and to share it with the world.

When I teach yoga classes, I always send my students home with "homework." I ask them, while sitting in easy cross legged pose after savasana to bring their hands to their hearts and feel into their souls and find just one significant thing they learned and felt in class that day. I ask them to connect with that lesson and how it feels in their body. I ask them then to activate it in their systems, remember it, and express it. Their homework is then to activate that lesson and energy several times a day and SHARE it with others. I expect them to apply what they have learned to their encounters out in the world, to influence others as they have been influenced by the yoga in my class. Then, I seal their practice with the blessing *namasté* and I explain to them that their homework is the essence of namasté, sharing the light in themselves in a way that they recognize and honor the light in others.

> *"What do you know about this business?"*
> *the King said to Alice.*
> *"Nothing," said Alice.*
> *"Nothing whatever?" persisted the King.*
> *"Nothing whatever," said Alice.*
> *"That's very important," the said, turning to the jury. They were just beginning to write this down on their slates when the White Rabbit interrupted: "Unimporant, you Majesty means, of course," he said in a very respectful tone, but frowning and making faces at him as he spoke. "Unimportant, of course, I meant," the King hastily said, and when ton to himself in an undertone, "important—unimportant—unimportant—important"*

As the trial progresses, the evidence offered by the testimonies of witnesses seems increasingly irrelevant to the case. When Alice is called to the stand, the King even announces that her testimony is unimportant, but not before he accidentally calls it very important. The Knave may or may not have stolen the Queen's tarts, and the evidence in the trial seems entirely unimportant, rendering the trial itself rather useless.

For Alice, and for anyone else who experiences a trial, a tribulation, a challenge, a trauma or a tragedy in life, the process of the challenge can seem very senseless. However, the experience of the trial is far from unimportant. Rather it has a tremendous impact on everyone involved. As with everything else in Wonderland, the entire trial process of gathering and testifying evidence makes absolutely no sense to Alice. However, the experience of it has great meaning as it has changed her at depth. Any trial, tribulation, trauma or tragedy of life has great meaning because the mere experience of it changes us at depth. We are different and cannot ever go back to the way we used to be.

"If there's no meaning in it," said the King, "that saves a world of trouble, you know, as we needn't try to find any."

After Alice's testimony, the White Rabbit presents an unsigned letter into evidence. Taking the letter as proof of the Knave's guilt, the Queen demands a sentence before a verdict is rendered. Alice expresses her disgust with the proceedings, that a sentence should not take place until after the verdict. She points out that the note reads that the stolen tarts are returned, thus obliterating the charge and purpose for the trial. The Queen orders Alice to be executed, but Alice, having grown to her full size, screams in anger, deeming the whole community as "nothing but a pack of cards." The cards go flying everywhere, symbolic of the nonsense of Wonderland, and Alice awakens from her Wonderland dream, back on the river bank, with her head in her sister's lap, awakened from her dream of Wonderland.

Like the Wonderland's Moral Duchess, and all the characters' efforts in the Wonderland trial over the stolen tarts, we try every day to make sense of the non-sense of life. We try to find the meaning and purpose in the tragedies such as when a hurricane crashes into New Orleans, or a tsunami damages a nuclear power plant, or terrorists fly airplanes through buildings, or gunmen shoot up innocent people in public places. How do we understand the importance of such destruction? We launch investigations and put people on trial, but ultimately we are powerless to change what has already happened. And finding meaning in senseless acts is as pointless as holding a trial over stolen tarts that were never really stolen.

We can, however, acknowledge and recognize how the event or encounter has changed us. What does hold meaning is how we respond to tragedy, and how we choose to live our lives as a result. We can step into our true power, our spiritual power, and control that which is entirely in our control, how we react to things.

Just as Alice stands up in her full-size when the Queen orders her to be executed, we can stand up for our own Truths by making choices that match our Truth and are important to us, allowing anything that is unimportant to come tumbling down like a house of cards. The King and

Queen of Hearts were seated on their throne when they arrived, with a great crowd assembled about them—all sorts of little birds and beasts, as well as the whole pack of cards: the Knave was standing before them, in chains, with a soldier on each side to guard him; and near the King was the White Rabbit, with a trumpet in one hand, and a scroll of parchment in the other.

5-Minute Practice Overview
Final Rest

I am focused and clear.
I am open to insight and intuition.

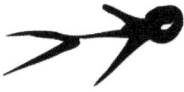 Savasana

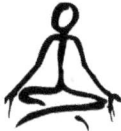 Namaste

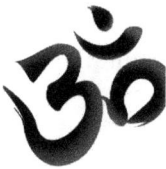 OM

Savasana

ASANA

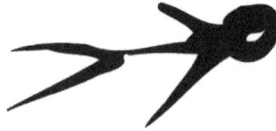

INTENTION

My work is done.
I enjoy the fruits of my labor.
I am open to receiving blessings.
I take in life fully and naturally.
I am serene.

Namasté

ASANA

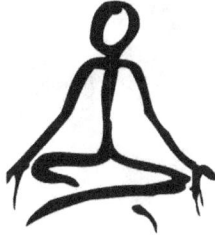

INTENTION

I am receptive to the wisdom and healing of Spirit.
I accept the healing and wisdom given to me.
I fill my mind with the wisdom of Spirit.
I fill my heart with the energy of Spirit.
I am grateful
My practice is affirmed and sealed.

OM

ASANA

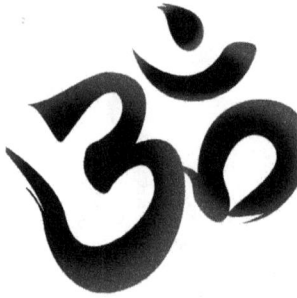

INTENTION

I am humble and honor the Divine in everything.
I am empty and complete.
I am connected through tissue and bone to the energy of sound.
I feel the vibration through the cavern of my being.
Energy is created.
Energy is sustained.
Energy is destroyed.
My process is complete and ready to be reborn.

Off the Mat Trick
MOZI Method – AJNA

Benefits

ASANA - open and clear neurological pathways
INTENTION -focused thoughts and clarity
SPIRIT -ability to see both the big picture and small details

ASANA - MOVE

- Gaze at the horizon to take in the big picture landscape
- Focus on one point
- Switch your vision from big picture to fine focus with breath

INTENTION - THINK

- "I am focused and clear"
- "I see the big picture"
- "I manage details without losing the big picture perspective"

SPIRIT - BREATHE

Breathe in as focus on one point
Breathe out as you gaze at the big picture landscape

Dosage

Practice this 1-3 x a day for 5-10 breaths

- 10 breaths when you wake up
- 5 breaths when you are driving long distances
- 10 breaths before getting into bed

Seated Final Rest
Journal

Date/Time:

Mood
> Body -
> Mind -
> Spirit -

Intention

Practice Summary

Insight

Alice's Evidence

Enlightenment
Waking from the Dream

Such a Curious Dream

"Oh, I've had such a curious dream!" said Alice, and she told her sister, as well as she could remember them, all these strange Adventures of hers that you have just been reading about; and when she had finished, her sister kissed her, and said, "It was a curious dream dear, certainly: but now run in to your tea; it's getting late." So Alice got up and ran off, thinking while she ran, as well she might, what a wonderful dream it had been.

At the end of *Alice's Adventures in Wonderland,* Alice awakes in the lap of her sister. The falling cards of Wonderland transformed into falling leaves from the trees. While Alice's older sister recognizes that Alice's adventures were just a dream, Alice's imagination allows her to hold onto her Adventures with curiosity.

Many yogis seek *enlightenment* which is that awareness of Spirit the extends beyond the every mundanity of life. What Alice and her Adventures in Wonderland teach us is that one of the easiest and most pleasurable ways to access the wonders and curiosity of Spirit is through imagination.

When I first started practicing yoga, my teachers taught me to visualize things happening within my body. One of the most memorable classes I ever took was when a teacher encouraged me to actually become the shapes I was forming in my body. She insisted that yoga was the most exhilarating experience of her life because she got to climb mountains, soar like an eagle, become a tree, and illuminate her world like a half-moon. The "pretending" aspect of yoga helped me to remember the vibrant life I had as a child in my make-believe worlds.

. . .and still as she listened, or seemed to listen, the whole place around her became alive with the strange creatures of her little sister's dream.
So she sat on, with closed eyes, and half believed herself in Wonderland, though she knew she had but to open them again and all would change to dull reality—the grass would be only rustling in the wind, the pool rippling to the waving of the reeds—the rattling teacups would

change to tinkling sheep-bells, and the Queen's shrill cries to the voice of the shepherd boy—and the sneeze of the baby, the shriek of the Gryphon, and all the other queer noises, would change (she knew) to the confused glamour of the busy farm-yard—while the lowing of the cattle in the distance would take the place of the Mock Turtle's heavy sobs.

After Alice runs off to tea, her sister stays in the farm-yard and takes a moment to close her eyes and "pretend" that she is in Alice's Wonderland. She quickly recognizes how the mundane sounds the farmyard informed Alice's dream, and that with just a little imagination, simple things can be truly wondrous.

Our dream-world comes alive when our mundane world sleeps, just as our mundane world comes alive when our dream-world sleeps. The ultimate *waking* is when we recognize, acknowledge, and allow the two worlds to blend, unite, and merge. When Alice's sister hears that the sounds of the farmyard blended into the mystical land of Alice's wonderland, she *woke* to the power of the imagination to make-believe magic out of the mundane.

As children, we are encouraged to play in the world of make-believe. But somewhere in the process of adolescence and rites of passage into adulthood, our capacity to play in wonder and curiosity is squelched by the "reality" of the mundane. As yogis, when we fall onto our mats in Child's Pose, we are encouraged to allow ourselves to go back to the child's mind, and activate our latent imaginations and exercise the atrophied muscles of make-believe.

Perhaps, the phrase "make-believe" is just that, a world that we Make by Believing. When I swing my arms into eagle pose and fan my toes like tail feathers in crow pose, I Make myself Believe for that moment that I have the abilities of an eagle or a crow. When I do that, insights strike me, and I get ideas and wisdoms I never could conceive if I stayed in the world of the mundane. In that make-believe world, I expand the possibilities of my reality, and stretch my perceptions beyond the mundane.

Lastly, she pictured to herself how this same little sister of hers would, in the after-time, be herself a grown woman; and how she would keep, through all her riper years, the simple and loving heart of her childhood: and how she would gather about her other little children, and make their eye bright and eager with many a strange tale, perhaps even with the dream of Wonderland long-ago.

Grateful that Alice has helped her access imagination again, Alice's sister hopes that as Alice becomes a grown woman, she not only stays in touch with the world of Wonderland, but she is able to help other children keep it alive in themselves.

Wonderland lives INSIDE us. So many yogis have been taught to believe that to reach *enlightenment* is a long-enduring process. But the truth is that we all have moments of *wokeness* all the time, we simply need to acknowledge those moments for what they are.

When we live in the moment, allow ourselves to Make-Believe them into bigger vaster experiences, we awaken our most abundant resource, IMAGINATION, and our world becomes limitless.

The White Rabbit Hops Away

In yoga and in life, the best teachers are those like Alice's White Rabbit. Not because they show you all the twists and turns of the rabbit hole tunnels, but because they hop away. They lock the doors to their classes once you learned their lessons. They abandon you. They leave you to find your way through yourself. The best teachers expect that you learned what they had to teach and leave you to find your own way with your acquired skills.

We call that graduation.

Somewhere along my own ventures in Yoga Wonderland, I allowed my imagination to open up wide like a telescope. I believe so much in Yoga Wonderland and all the adventures that happen there that I hung up my white rabbit waistcoat and threw away my timepiece, shutting the door to the dark yoga rabbit holes behind me. In November of 2018, I retired from teaching public yoga classes and workshops. That's when I decided I wanted to be an owl in Yoga Wonderland, and I got myself a crooked purple mortar board and a strawberry flavored tootsie pop. Cuz here in wonderland, *why lick the tootsie pop when we can chew!* As the tootsie-pop owl, your not-white-rabbit, I refuse to be a main character in your yoga story. Because, that's not what wonderland is about!

Wonderland is about looking INSIDE YOURSELF.
YOU are the main character in your story.

YOGA WONDERLAND

www.ingramcontent.com/pod-product-compliance
Lightning Source LLC
Chambersburg PA
CBHW071210090426
42736CB00014B/2771